Come Home, Daddy: An Early-Onset Alzheimer's Memoir

April Enciso

Preface

After my father's death in 2018, I decided I wanted to share my experiences of his battle with Alzheimer's to try to help others with the disease, as well as their caregivers. When my father was diagnosed in 2014, my mom and I had no knowledge of how the disease would progress, including what my dad would go through and what we would experience as caregivers.

In this book, I want to share not only my dad's fight with Alzheimer's, but also a few of the strategies we used to deal with some of his challenging behavior in the disease's later stages. Alzheimer's is not just a disease where you forget people and things. In my dad's case, he developed a different personality from the one he had before. My dad used to be a headstrong, stubborn, independent person, but he became a dependent person, often sad and crying. At the end, he experienced hallucinations, made inappropriate comments, became increasingly agitated and hostile. When we could no longer care for him at home, we put him in a nursing home. At thirty-nine years of age, I never thought I would have to put one of my parents into a nursing home when he was only sixty-seven.

I wrote this book from my point of view as his daughter, but I wasn't present for all of the conversations. Where I have written about these discussions and events, I have based them on what family and friends told me occurred. Some names, locations, and identifying characteristics have been changed to protect the privacy of those depicted. Dialogue has been recreated from memory.

Chapter One

The Store

It was a slow day at the store. My dad, Wendell, and Uncle Jimmy were gathered around the front counter playing poker. My father, David, was a tall man at six-foot-one, medium build, with skin that was moderately tanned from being out in the sun. He had a dark brown beard and mustache and blue-green eyes that today were accentuated by his shirt: a Western-style, blue-and-purple, long-sleeve plaid shirt with snaps over dark indigo-blue Levis. He also wore black sneakers and a blue ball cap over his curly brown hair that said "Surplus and Salvage Sales, Inc." This was my father's standard wardrobe. He never preferred to wear shirts with buttons.

Wendell stood beside him. He was shorter than my father, and his build was a slimmer with a light tan complexion that was somewhat concealed by his glasses. Wendell was in his seventies with graying hair, and working at my dad's business was his second career in life, after working for the United States Postal service as a mail carrier. He was also a preacher and, surprisingly, had a bit of a mischievous side.

Uncle Jimmy stood across from them, medium height with a slim build, wearing gray-rimmed glasses that accentuated the gray hair that thinned on the top of his head. He wore a long-sleeve red dress shirt with a pair of black slacks and dress shoes. The majority of my father's uncles and aunts preferred to wear dressier clothing. Uncle Jimmy was actually my dad's uncle, but everyone just called him Uncle Jimmy, including Wendell. Uncle Jimmy was known for carrying liquor in a mouthwash bottle to disguise it and bringing it to work at the store. Sometimes, Uncle Jimmy would take naps on the job, propping his feet up on the desk and going to sleep when they weren't busy. Then, finding him sleeping, Wendell would give Uncle Jimmy what he called "The Hot Foot." Wendell would light a match and place it between the sole and heel of Uncle Jimmy's shoe. Uncle Jimmy would awaken hastily and have some choice things to tell Wendell each and every time.

A stream of smoke blew towards them from my dad's cigarette in the nearby ashtray. My dad dealt out five cards to Wendell, Uncle Jimmy, and himself. They checked and raised in a round, playing with my dad's poker set, full of red, white, and blue chips. When my family played with poker chips, white represented one dollar, blue five dollars, and the red chip ten dollars. My dad had just bet five dollars, and it was down to Wendell and Jimmy to decide if they'd call or fold. They called in tandem and placed one blue chip each on the table. Since they were playing draw poker, each player could trade up to three cards during their turn.

With a concerned look on his face Wendell said, "I'd like to trade two cards, please." He discarded two of his cards, and my dad dealt him two new ones. Expressionless, Uncle Jimmy followed by requesting three cards.
"I'll take one card," said Dad.
Wendell checked, and Uncle Jimmy raised, making Wendell yell out with a flabbergasted look on his face, "I fold!" My dad raised again, and Uncle Jimmy called, placing an additional blue chip on the table.
Now that the round of betting was complete, Uncle Jimmy laid down his hand: three nines, a king, and a jack. But when my dad laid down his hand, he had a full house: three queens and two fives.
Uncle Jimmy cursed in disappointment. "Oh crap, I thought you were bluffing and had nothing!" My dad often did bluff well during poker games. Even when he didn't have a good hand his face would remain stoic. His opponents would fold, and he would win the pot of money.
"You won again! Are you counting cards, David?" Wendell asked with a smirk on his face.
"No, of course not!" my dad said. "Hey, you're lucky we're playing with poker chips, or you'd owe me real money!"
Outside the window a blue pickup truck was visible pulling into the parking lot and parking. "Back to work," said my dad.

~~~

"The Store," that's the name my family gave my dad's flooring business, Surplus and Salvage Sales, Inc. My dad sold carpet, vinyl, carpet pad, wood flooring, and miscellaneous building supplies such as windows and doors. The store was in a run-down area of town called Millville. It was mostly industrial buildings, but there were some older homes in the area. "The Store" consisted of several buildings that were not in great shape: all of them needed repairs and new roofs, and there were several leaks we had to put buckets under to catch water droplets when it rained. There were four buildings total: the front office that held my dad's and his younger brother Uncle Mark's desks, the secretary's office, and most importantly the Store's only AC unit and bathroom. The front office was where they wrote up all the "tickets," or invoices, for customer purchases. Nothing was
~~~

computerized except the credit card machine. Then there was a large warehouse where they stored all the carpet, carpet pad, vinyl, and some of the windows and doors.   My cousin Shannon and I used to play in the warehouse when we were young, running and jumping on the giant carpet rolls. It probably wasn't the safest thing to do, but we had fun.

The third building was one my Uncle Mark used for his woodworking business. Most commonly he took orders for custom kitchen cabinets, but sometimes he would make furniture such as bookcases.   We were not allowed in that building due the equipment he had in there, including several large saws. There was however, a swampy area right behind it that had water and lily pads. My father had seen several snakes in the pond, so we weren't allowed to go there either.

The fourth building in actuality should have been condemned, and at the time of this poker game, I hadn't been it in since I was a child. When we were children, my cousin Shannon and I would play with a Cowboys and Indians board game in there. A few years after, the roof gave out and rainwater leaked into the building. Now the building is contaminated with mold, and the roof is falling in.

With the business being in a bad area of town, some homeless people came into the Store asking for food or money. They never left empty-handed. My father would take them to the local grocery store called Piggy Wiggly and get them a boxed lunch or take them to Jimmy's Drive-In and get them a box of fried chicken.

My father insisted on feeding all the employees lunch every day, too. He would buy them lunch from one of the local businesses—I remember many times while I worked there getting permission to go up to Jimmy's Drive Through and pick up lunch for everyone—or he would cook extra food the night before to bring in so everyone would be able to eat.

He treated everyone there fairly and considered all the employees family. Over the holidays, he would host a Christmas lunch at the Store for our family, friends, and customers. Anyone was welcome to come, and to invite others, too! My father would get premade ham, vegetables, and rolls from the Piggy Wiggly. I remember sometimes we would be close to running out of food, and he would send someone or himself up to that Piggy Wiggly to get more food to make sure we would have enough.

~~~

In his youth, my dad was a master poker and pool player. He used to stay out late at night playing at the Elks club or various bars with his father. He made good money doing this, but my mother didn't like him staying out all night and drinking.
~~~

I remember one time when I was a child, my mother woke me in the middle of the night. My mother, Renee, was wearing a T-shirt and blue jeans, her long, dark brown hair parted in the middle and styled. Her smoky gray eye shadow emphasized her brown eyes. She was petite and always looked younger than she really was. I remember thinking it was odd she was dressed and not in her pajamas.

She picked me up, took me outside to the backseat of her silver Oldsmobile, and buckled me in.

"Where are we going, Mommy?" I asked, sleepily.

My mother responded with a displeased look on her face, "We are going to go get your father."

After ten minutes we arrived at our destination, and we headed into a small building. We were at a bar, it was very dark, and cigarette smoke flowed freely through the room. We headed to the pool table where my father was. I remember some older man saying as we passed, "That child shouldn't be in here." My mother ignored him.

Upon reaching the pool table, my mother said in a stern voice, "David, you need to come home it's late."

"Come home, Daddy," I added in a timid voice.

Looking at us, my father relented, and we all left together.

My mother in the coming months made an agreement with my father that he could drink as much as he wanted, but at home. She was worried he'd kill someone or himself drunk driving. Growing up, I remember him often drinking a twelve-pack of beer a night and smoking a pack of cigarettes every day, and I believe this contributed to the many cardiovascular issues he had later in life.

But even after my father stopped going out to bars and the Elks Lodge he still liked to play poker. We played poker at home often as a family. He also had a handheld poker game and a PlayStation One poker game he played. He would play the games for hours and carry the handheld poker game with him to work. Shortly before we realized something was going on with his memory, he stopped playing them both. At the time, we thought he had just lost interest, but perhaps he had forgotten how to play.

Chapter Two

Childhood Memories

My father, David, was born on May 28, 1950, in a small town called Panama City, Florida. He lived with his parents until they separated. His mother left when he was five and his brother was a baby. After that, he lived with his paternal grandparents at their house through high school. His younger brother, Mark, who was an infant at the time of separation, went to live with his maternal grandparents.

Both David's paternal grandfather and grandmother were fantastic role models. His grandfather, whom he called "Papaw," was a preacher and started his own church, First United Pentecostal. Papaw was a tall man, with white-gray hair and silver glasses. He was always happy when I saw him as a child. He used to do a trick where he would show me his dentures and then take them out to make it look like he had no teeth. He usually dressed in suits or finely tailored dress clothes.

My father's grandmother, "Mamaw," was the matriarch of the house, always organizing everything and taking care of everyone. She was on the shorter side, with solid white hair accentuated by her silver glasses. She wove her hair tightly into a bun on top of her head every day.

I remember one particular story he would tell me about driving with Papaw. My father was in the backseat with his cousin, and Papaw would turn around, talking to them both, and not pay attention to driving! After having a long conversation with them he turned back around to the front and saw a car in front of him was stopped, so he slammed on breaks and said, "Crazy woman." The person in front of him had probably stopped at a normal pace, but since he was talking to them in the backseat he had no clue. Many of my family members say he used to have an angel looking over him because he did things like that all the time and never got in a wreck!

David met my mother in 1973, and they got married in 1975. Three years later, I was born, and would remain an only child.

My parents moved to Panama City so my father could help my grandfather, David Jr., with his business. Like his parents, my grandfather also wore silver-rimmed glasses with greying hair, and was overweight with a larger frame. He generally wore polo shirts and dress slacks. David Jr. was my grandfather, and I called him "Papaw" as well. Papaw took my cousin, Shannon, and me to do lots of fun things on the weekend: horseback riding, the circus, and shopping to name a few.

Shannon was two years younger than me, so she was always slightly shorter and had beautiful, curly blond hair. Shannon was like my sister growing up: we were both only children and would get to play together during the summers at my house, either in the pool or with Barbies in the two-story dollhouse my father built me. Another of our favorite activities was making movies with a video camera Shannon had. We'd play anywhere we could with the video camera, including at the store while Papaw was checking the books.

In 1999, we found out Papaw had lung cancer. He was a lifelong smoker and had had a pacemaker inserted for a heart condition a few years before. The tumor in his lung was directly behind the pacemaker, so it wasn't noticed until it was too late. The cancer spread to his bones, then his brain. I thought this would motivate my father to stop smoking and perhaps stop drinking, but it didn't. When we broached the subject of quitting smoking with him after my grandfather's death, my father said, "Well, I've got to die from something."

He inherited the Surplus and Salvage Sales, Inc. business from his father in 1999 when he passed away.

~~~

Throughout my childhood, I remember my father working long hours at the Store. It was open Monday through Saturday, and Saturday was a half-day. They closed at 5:00 p.m. Monday through Friday, but my father would often stay late if he had customers come in right before he closed.

Sometimes Dad would close the Store and we would go to the beach at Cape San Blas. Back then you could drive your vehicle right up on the sand. As a kid, I thought that was pretty cool. The beach looked immaculate even though it had been driven on. You could see the car tire tracks on the glistening white sand. We'd always bring coolers with drinks and pick up a Church's Fried Chicken bucket on the way there. We'd set up chairs and eat the chicken on the beach while sitting in the sunshine. It wasn't always sunny, though. In the summer afternoon showers would come on quickly, and we would get into the truck and wait for it to pass. We sat through many thunderstorms in my dad's Bronco truck. He had a massive wrench connected to the front of the Bronco, and many times I watched him pull his friends or people that he didn't know out of the wet sand at the beach. It was sometimes hard to tell whether specific areas could be driven on.
~~~

We went bowling on the weekends a lot, too, at a bowling alley called Hickory Lanes. During nighttime bowling hours, they had something called *twilight bowling* where they turned out all the lights and a disco ball would spin, lighting all the bowling lanes. We'd generally arrive in the afternoon, sometimes to meet up with my parents' friends. Once there, my mother and I would either bowl with my dad and their friends or go hang out in the arcade and play video games. My father was a great bowler: I remember sitting there watching him score strikes and spares. If you got three strikes in a row, you would get something called a turkey, and on the monitor a picture of a turkey would display.

When I was a smaller child, my father also took me fishing. I still have my child-size fishing rod that he bought me. My parents said I liked to fish and play with the worms they used as bait. I do not fish now, but it was something fun to do with my parents when I was a kid. My father had the first fish I caught stuffed and put on the wall alongside his own prized catches.

One memory in particular will always stay with me. It was the day my father saved our lives. I was probably around five or six years old. We were driving in my dad's green pickup truck, I don't recall where, but it was a two-lane highway. The driver on the other side of the road was overtaking other cars and having a difficult time getting back in. My mother was freaking out because the car was headed straight for us in our lane. My father's face remained stoic. He drove onto the shoulder to get out of the way of the oncoming vehicle, and the car passed by. If my father hadn't driven onto the shoulder, we would have hit the car head on. His quick thinking saved us that day.

While I was still going to high school, my father let me work for him at the Store. I did the accounting and manned the front desk, answering the phone. Working there was my first experience with accounting before taking an accounting class in college. I balanced the books and wrote all the checks for the bills that needed to be paid for the business, though my father was very good at math as well. They used paper invoices for his business, so everything was handwritten. Dad would manually add, subtract, multiply, or divide without using a calculator. He could do the math for the fractions all in his head.

He let me work part-time doing this, so he had another employee fill in the gaps and train me. He continued to allow me to work for him part-time as I went to community college. At the time, I felt lucky to be able to work there with my family, to earn money and learn a new skill. I didn't realize until much later how much my father did for me.

The business did well while I was growing up. We weren't rich, but we weren't poor either. I always had everything I needed, and we had a little extra to buy things we wanted. My father paid for both my community college tuition and then my university college when I moved to Pensacola and attended University of West Florida (UWF). He bought my first three cars, a Camaro (which I stupidly wrecked as a sixteen-year-old), a Nissan 200SX, and a Ford Thunderbird. I realize now how fortunate I was, and that many parents would or can't afford to do these things for their children.

Chapter Three

My Father and His Mother

When I moved to Pensacola, my future husband (also named David) would often come back home with me on the weekends to see my parents. We would visit for holidays like Christmas, Thanksgiving, Easter, and birthdays.

David and I had dated briefly in high school and got back together after he finished college. He was short and had a stocky, muscular build, with dark brown skin, a stubble beard, and jet-black hair and eyes. David is originally from Colombia and came to the States when he was eight years old. After he finished college, he moved with me to Pensacola so I could finish my bachelor's degree in Computer Information Systems at UWF, where I later obtained my master's degree in Computer Science.

My contact with my father lessened during this time, since we didn't live in the same house or work together anymore. My mother would call me daily, so I would talk to her on the phone and sometimes talk to my dad, but Dad just wasn't the kind of person to call and speak to you every day. I'm that way too.

A few years before this time we learned that my Grandmother Nelle (my father's mother) had early-onset dementia. Since we didn't talk to her, we had no insight into the progression of her disease or any other related information. We just knew his mother had early-onset dementia and that there was a possibility my dad would get it, too.

The only memory I have of my grandmother is the one and only time I visited her as a child. I was around eight years old, and we went to her house in Drayton, South Carolina. It was very luxurious. She had remarried, and she and her husband were very well off. She was a gorgeous woman—her brown hair and makeup were perfectly set, and she wore a patterned silk blouse and black dress slacks. They had a two-story house, and I remember playing on the staircase, which was probably not advisable since I was not supervised.

My grandmother invited me into her room to show me her jewelry. She took out her jewelry box, and I looked at the precious objects inside. I was in awe—there was so much! Each piece had huge gemstones, probably around two carats for several of the pieces. She took out an emerald and ruby set of earrings.

"You can have these if you like them," she said smiling. I thanked her excitedly and took the earrings with me.

Later that night, everyone was playing card games. After a while, my mother took me upstairs so I could sleep. The next thing I remember is being awakened by my mother saying we were leaving right then, in the middle of the night. My dad and my grandmother had had an argument that led to my dad saying we were all leaving immediately. My mother told me we weren't taking the emerald and ruby earrings, and so I reluctantly left them there. I never saw my grandmother again after that. My father didn't speak to her again. The only correspondence we had with her was through a card when I graduated from community college. That was when we found out from her husband that she had dementia.

In 2016, my mother was able to find my dad's half-sister on Facebook. We found out that my grandmother first started showing symptoms at age fifty-two and died at age seventy-six.

Based on my research, having a first-degree relative with Alzheimer's increases your risk of developing it. Early-onset Alzheimer's, which develops before age sixty, is linked to inheriting a mutated gene. A parent has a fifty-percent chance of passing the gene to their offspring. Late-onset Alzheimer's, which occurs after age sixty-five, has been linked to the APOE e4 gene, which can also be inherited from your parents, but having the gene doesn't necessarily mean you will get it.

I feel like my grandmother and my father both having dementia and Alzheimer's was related; it's possible he inherited the gene from her.

Chapter Four

First Sign Of Trouble

In 2010, my mother called to let me know that some of my dad's coworkers had told her he was asking the same questions over and over again and that they were having repeated conversations. My dad was unaware that he was doing this, and when questioned about it by my mom he denied repeating himself. This behavior went on for a while, and then an incident occurred at work with his secretary saying he said something inappropriate to her. He denied saying anything inappropriate, and we thought maybe she was making it up. It wasn't until later that we realized that saying inappropriate things—even things in the wrong context or time in a conversation—was part of Alzheimer's, so it's very possible my father did say something inappropriate and didn't remember doing it. The secretary ended up sending my father a certified letter about the inappropriate comment. My father signed for the letter, read it, then shredded it and put it in the garbage. Even after receiving the certified letter, he denied that the incident happened. The secretary quit right after that in 2011.

His coworker Wendell continued to be concerned about the repeated conversations. Shortly after that, my dad began not being able to write ticket invoices anymore. He could no longer perform math calculations in his head either. There was a TV in the office where my dad had his desk. He began coming to work, going straight to the office, and sitting at his desk watching TV. He would remain there all day until it was time to go home, then he would leave. We knew something was going on at this point but didn't know it was Alzheimer's.

My mom pleaded with my dad to get tested. He refused and said nothing was wrong, that he wasn't having memory issues. I feel like my father may have known something was wrong and didn't want to go to the doctor. He was quick-witted and intelligent, and we think for a long time he found ways to hide what was going on until the symptoms became noticeable to others. Even when he had progressed much further, he would still try to hide it when asked questions by the doctor. The doctor would ask him,

"What day is it today?" and he would say, "I don't need to know what day it is, I'm retired!"

My parents would sometimes drive over to Pensacola to see my husband and I. My father always drove them, as my mother does not like to drive. In 2012, though, he began having noticeable issues driving. As my mother directed him on which way to turn, he would not turn when he needed to. He was probably starting to have trouble comprehending at this point, or his comprehension of the directions she was giving him was delayed.

There is one specific incident in the early days of his life with Alzheimer's that I will always remember: I had been in the hospital for the birth of my first child, Eva, and my husband had coincidently been admitted to the hospital right after Eva's birth due to an infected bite from our cat, Pumma.

Pumma was a large shorthaired tabby, solid black with green eyes. Pumma was a strange cat, in that he liked to play fetch with his toy balls and he enjoyed eating plastic, so we always equated him to a dog for these preferences. One time while we were out of town, he skinned his mouse toy, ate the skin, ate the plastic, then puked part of the plastic up on our bed. He was an interesting cat, to say the least.

In a rush, my husband had gone home to grab our hospital bag. We hadn't taken it with us when I first went to the hospital; I didn't think I would be admitted since I wasn't in labor at that time. We always kept the doors to the bedrooms shut so the cat dander wouldn't get in, as I am mildly allergic and wasn't sure if the new baby would be as well. As my husband opened the door to the baby's room to grab the bag, Pumma darted in.

My husband grabbed Pumma to take him out, but he unfortunately got him on his back, where Pumma had arthritis. He'd even had several steroid shots over the years to help with the pain. So Pumma turned around and bit my husband's hand. In a rush to get back to the hospital, my husband cleaned the bite, put a liquid Band-Aid on it to seal it, and returned to the hospital. The wound got infected, and right after my daughter was born, he was admitted to the hospital. He ended up having to have surgery to drain the wound since it had become so infected and inflamed.

Since my husband was still in the hospital when I was discharged, my mother would drive us home. My father was going to follow my mom, Eva, and I in his truck. My mom and I got into my car, and my dad got into his truck. But before my mom could pull out to get in front of him, my dad started driving. We have no idea where he is going—and I'm sure he didn't either!

"Where is he going?" I asked my mother.

Surprised she said, "I have no idea, I told him to wait until we get in front of him!"

He continued to drive off, crossing traffic, and went across the street to park in a shopping mall's parking lot. At that point, I can only assume he realized he had no clue where he was going and stopped. My mom and I drove over to where he was at the mall and parked next to him.

"You were supposed to follow us. Why did you start driving?" she asked him.

"I don't know," he replied.

After that, he got behind us and followed us to my house, but both my mom and I knew something was very wrong. My dad had always been an excellent and confident driver, and it wasn't like him to get lost.

~~~

Things at the business continued to decline. When my grandfather ran the company, he would always come in on the weekends and check the books. I remember this well because Sunday was my cousin Shannon's and my day to be with our grandfather. We would play games at the Store while he was reviewing the books. My grandfather was doing this to make sure whatever secretary they had at the time was not stealing money, and that everything checked out. Once my grandfather passed away, my dad never did these types of checks that we are aware of.

So, in 2013, we found out that one of the secretaries had been embezzling a great deal of money from the business. Instead of paying the bills to the carpet suppliers, she had been writing checks to a third-party account. By the time we realized she had stolen the money, she had quit, and no one could find her.

We found out after the fact that she was convicted and charged with stealing from another business she worked for after she had worked for my father. When they searched her car, the police found payroll worksheets from my father's business for two of his employees.

At this point, my father's personality started to change. Before the personality changes, he had enjoyed coming home from work and going out to the shed he built to hang out in with his two dogs. He had made a homemade smoker that he used to grill us delicious steaks. He was a master griller, and we had enjoyed all kinds of grilled foods when I was growing up: steaks, hamburgers, chicken, sausage, and pork chops. I always looked forward to what he cooked. Then, right before bed, he would come into the house to tell my mother goodnight.
~~~

But when the personality changes began, he stopped hanging out with the dogs as much. He would come into the house earlier and sit at the kitchen table while my mother was cooking dinner. My mother thought that he was hungry and coming in early for that reason, but now we believe he just wanted to be with her. Where he was once independent and wanted to be alone, he was now more dependent and sought out company. Around this time was when he also stopped playing his beloved handheld poker game. He began crying for no reason that was obvious to us. We realized later in his progression that this was all just part of the disease.

Chapter Five

Trying to Get a Diagnosis

In 2014, my father saw a neurologist in Panama City who diagnosed him with Alzheimer's disease with mild cognitive decline. He was prescribed Namenda XR 28 mg for Alzheimer's. Namenda XR doesn't stop the disease, but it slows its progression. I was happy to finally have a diagnosis for what was going on and that there was some treatment available.

However, it had taken a long time to get a diagnosis because my mother's insurance would initially only pay for a CT scan of my father's brain, and the CT scan didn't show anything abnormal. The doctor told us that a PET scan is more commonly used for an Alzheimer's diagnosis. After fighting the insurance company for a few months, they were finally able to get a PET scan authorized. The PET scan was consistent with findings of Alzheimer's disease: it showed he had decreased uptake in the parietal and mesial temporal lobes, which is commonly seen in Alzheimer's disease. The MRI that was done at the same time noted he had atrophy in the central and cortical areas of the brain.

The issues at the Store continued as my father was not able to work. My mom worked as a paraprofessional at Cedar Grove Elementary School at the time. Sometimes during the summer, she would work at the business to help my dad out, mainly when they were in between secretaries. In the summer of 2014, she took up her post as usual, and that's when she realized he was doing nothing except watching TV.

Seeing it daily, in person, my mother realized my father needed to retire, as he couldn't work anymore. She helped him get everything ready to close the business, and they paid the outstanding bills the business had. Then they went to the Social Security office to apply for Social Security Disability. After multiple tries, they got his doctor to write a letter stating that he had Alzheimer's. His Social Security Disability application was finally approved, so he began receiving payments from the federal government. Since he was only sixty-three at the time, he didn't qualify for regular Social Security yet. After that, my mother went to see a lawyer friend and got papers drawn up to so that she had power of attorney for my dad.

After he retired, my father stayed home and didn't go anywhere, as he could no longer drive. He would watch TV all day, and my mom would leave lunch for him to heat up in the microwave.

Over the next few years, my father continued to have other health issues in addition to his Alzheimer's diagnosis. From a young age, my father had smoked cigarettes, and had drunk quite a lot for as long as I could remember. Later in 2014, he started to have severe leg pain, pain so severe he could not walk for extended periods because of it. After having an ultrasound of his legs, we found out he had Peripheral Artery Disease (PAD), which meant that the major veins in his legs had a blockage. In January 2015, he had stents placed in both legs, but after the surgery, he was still having pain in his left leg. Upon further investigation, the doctor determined the stent had not taken and the vein was still blocked, so in March 2015, he had another surgery called femoropopliteal bypass surgery so that his blood could go around the blocked artery. The surgery was a success, and he did not have the severe leg pain anymore, but the doctor put him on blood thinner medication.

In March 2015, my dad had a bowel movement with a blood clot in it. By this time my mom was having to assist him with toileting, so she noticed and called the doctor immediately. The doctor told them to go to the ER to get it checked out. The ER doctor did a rectal exam and said he had a mass in the lower part of his rectum. The doctor admitted him to the hospital and scheduled a colonoscopy to examine the mass.

My mom called to tell me what was going on. I had just gotten my daughter Eva down for a nap, and I was attempting to take a nap since I had to be at the hospital at midnight to be induced for the birth of my second child, a boy we named Diego. The phone rang right as I was about to fall asleep, and I answered.

"Hello?"

"It's me," said my mother in an unsure voice. "The doctor at the ER said your father has a mass, and they want to do a colonoscopy in the morning to check out the mass. What should I do?"

"Go ahead and let them do the colonoscopy. The mass needs to be checked out to make sure it's not something bad," I said. I tried to keep it together for Mom, but upon hearing the news, I was worried, especially with the mass present, but I was hopeful it wasn't anything bad. My dad ended up getting admitted to the hospital for testing the next morning. It was a strange coincidence that another family member would again be in the hospital at the same time as I would be for my child's birth.

Immediately after the colonoscopy, the doctors scheduled an emergency surgery to remove the mass. The mass was sent off for testing, and it came back positive for cancer. Dad was officially diagnosed with rectal cancer in March 2015.

Over the next few weeks, he had a PET/CT scan to check if the cancer had metastasized to other areas of the body. The test indicated no evidence that it had spread. At that time, the doctor told Dad he needed to quit both smoking and drinking, which he did.

The doctor ordered both radiation and chemotherapy for treatment, then a follow-up surgery to cut out any of the remaining cancer cells that may have been left. My dad started radiation at Hope Radiation Cancer Center and was fitted for a chemo unit to wear at home. It was a little bag he wore over his shoulder that plugged the chemo unit into the PICC (Peripherally Inserted Central Catheter) line he had recently gotten. The PICC line was basically an IV that is inserted into a major vein in your chest or arm. Toxic medications such as chemo require a major vein because smaller veins may collapse. The chemo machine had a connection that plugged into his PICC line so it could dispense the medication throughout his body. Every week his chemo machine was preprogramed to dispense the medication at certain intervals. He received both chemo and radiation from April, 2015 to May 20, 2015.

When my dad got diagnosed with cancer, my mother had to retire early and quit her job as a paraprofessional. Even so, she struggled to deal with the combined pressures of my Dad's Alzheimer's disease and his cancer. It was a lot to handle on her own, though she did get help from Wendell, and he went to some of the radiation treatments with them. There was a Dairy Queen right next to the Hope Radiation Center, and every time they would go to get treatments my dad would say afterward that he needed to get ice cream. My mom would take him, and he always got a vanilla sundae. He really wasn't eating well during the chemo and radiation treatment, but he never turned down ice cream.

By the time my father completed his treatments, it had taken an enormous toll on his Alzheimer's. He had progressed into the moderate stage of the disease, and we think the combination of the chemo with the anesthesia for the surgeries made it worse. It appeared that every time he had to have any anesthesia afterward he would be in a brain fog that pushed him further along in the Alzheimer's progression.

Chapter Six

Moving Day

I convinced my mom that she and my dad needed to move to Pensacola, where I lived, so I could help take care of my dad and his declining health. We decided as soon as he finished his radiation and chemo treatments they would move, and then he would have the final surgery to remove any remaining rectal cancer.

My husband and I started searching for a house for them that was close to ours. We didn't find any pre-built houses in our price range that we liked, but we did find a new subdivision that had some lots available that we could build a house on. My parents came up and saw the house floor plan before we decided on the build. We closed on the house for them in March 2015, and we moved my parents up on May 28, my dad's sixty-fifth birthday.

My dad very vocally did not want to leave their house in Panama City, and he did have an adjustment period after they moved here. My dad, upon moving to the new, unfamiliar layout, started wandering around. He had problems locating the bathroom even though it was directly off the living room and in view, so he put a picture of a toilet on the door to help him locate it.

His primary care doctor got him an appointment for his final surgery with a rectal surgeon in Pensacola, Dr. Hudson. I accompanied my parents to the appointment. After waiting for a few minutes, the nurse led us to the exam room, which was rather large and had a long, tan countertop with cabinets on one side of the wall. Dr. Hudson entered. He was in his sixties, with graying hair, a medium build, and wore a loose-fitting shirt and pair of pants. We would learn that Dr. Hudson liked to golf just like my father, and my dad would often invite him to go with him sometime. While they never went, of course, my mother did take my dad to Scenic Hills Country Club's golf course, where Dr. Hudson liked to play.

That day, Dr. Hudson did an exam on my dad, and said, "He should have one more surgery to remove any cancerous cells that still exist. There are two options: the more preferred choice is that we remove the lower part of the rectum and fit him with a colostomy bag where the waste would go; the other option is to excise the area where the tumor was, but it may have side effects."

"I don't want to have the bag," my dad said immediately, and my mother wanted him to be happy, so we went with the second option.

~~~

My dad came through the surgery fine, and no more cancerous cells were found during the follow-up biopsy – all good news! However, his Alzheimer's did become worse after the surgery since he was put under anesthesia again. Afterward, he had the added side effect that, because the surgeons had to cut into the lower muscle in the rectum, his anal muscle did not always function correctly and couldn't always be controlled. This meant he would have accidents on occasion.

After having to throw out a few pairs of underwear and pants, my mom and I decided he would have to wear pull-up diapers. I went to the store and got him a box of pull-ups. We told him they were underwear and replaced all the real underwear in his dresser drawer with them, too. After a while, he accepted them as underwear, since he could no longer find the real underwear. They came in two colors, gray and blue. For some reason, the blue ones were the only acceptable ones in my father's eyes, so we went with those. We found out quickly after some leaking episodes that these pull-ups were not the best quality, and I found a better-quality pull-up diaper that we could order online. We tried them out: my dad was okay with them, and they worked a lot better and didn't leak as often.

By the time they moved to Pensacola, my dad was already at the point where he didn't know what day of the week it was. He always wanted to be with my mom, to the point where if she went to the bathroom he would wander around the house looking for her and calling her. He would follow her from room to room.

Around this time, he started hallucinating. We were lucky because most of his hallucinations were benign. They were usually focused on watching the TV: he would hallucinate that the people on TV were there in the house talking to him. He would come and let us know whoever was on the TV show was there, and that it was cool. We just nodded and said that was great. I found that as long as the hallucination was something positive and non-threating it was better for us to agree with him and that made him happy. Sometimes he would remember things incorrectly and tell us about it. Again, as long as it was not anything terrible, we would do the same thing, agree with him. Doing this kept him in a good mood and not agitated.

Since my dad had left pretty much all his friends in Panama City, he started getting bored staying at home after moving to Pensacola. He still wanted to do some of the things he had done before Alzheimer's, like
~~~

playing golf and going bowling. My mom would take him to play golf at Scenic Hills Country Club's golf course. At this point, he really couldn't play anymore, but he enjoyed the trip.

The increasing level of attention my dad needed was taking a toll on my mother, even though she had help from me. I read about something called respite care online and found a service that could help us. Once a week, the caregiver would take my father out bowling. I paid for this respite care for my dad. It was only four hours every Thursday, but it gave my mom time to herself that helped her.

My father's assigned caregiver was called Rodney, a tall man in his sixties. My dad liked that Rodney was close to his age. Rodney was a great person, and he cared a great deal for my father. They had a wonderful time together: they would dance to the music while bowling at the alley, and my dad looked forward to being with him every week.

My mom would send cash with my dad to pay for food, but she soon realized my dad was coming home with a lot less cash then he should. We don't know if someone was taking advantage of him not knowing how much money to pay for food or bowling, or whether he was handing cash out. She called and talked to the owner of the bowling alley, and they decided it would be okay for her to send a check from ten on.

My father started to experience *sundowning* around this time as well. Sundowning is a phenomenon where a person with Alzheimer's experiences confusion or agitation later in the day. To combat this, my mother avoided taking my father anywhere late in the day if possible. She also limited any visits to the house that were later in the day. She would close all window and door shades before the sun started to go down to help keep the light level constant in the house, and these techniques helped my father.

Chapter Seven

Paying for Nursing Home Care

By 2016, my dad had progressed to the point where he could no longer dress himself, and needed help with bathing and using the restroom. He required supervision at all times to instruct, guide him, and make sure he didn't try to leave the house.

At this point, my mother was getting extremely stressed, as she had to do almost everything except feed my dad because, at this point, he could still feed himself. It was similar to taking care of a small child. He would need instructions on simple things, like getting up from the chair to come to the table to eat, washing his hands, and using the toilet.

We started to consider putting him in a nursing home. While researching nursing homes, I realized the average cost per month for nursing home care in our area was $5,000 to $7,000. Neither my mom nor I realized it would be that expensive, and my parents didn't have much money. One of the reasons they moved up to Pensacola was for me to help them financially. The stock market crashed in 2008, before my dad had been diagnosed with Alzheimer's, and he had pulled all his money out of his retirement account and cashed it out. If he had left it in his accounts, it would have likely gained the losses back, but we think at that time he was starting to be affected and just made the wrong decision. In any case, they were living off the money that he had cashed out, as well as his social security payments.

I made an appointment with an elder law attorney to discuss possible options for paying for my dad's future nursing home care with Medicaid. My dad accompanied us to the meeting.

The lawyer's office was in Pensacola's historic downtown district, located in one of the older period homes. The building had old-fashioned wood flooring, and every room had dark wood crown molding with a unique design. The receptionist came to get us and led us to a room with a couch, two chairs, and a pool table.

"Nick will be with you shortly," she said as she pulled the two wooden doors closed.

Immediately, my dad was elated to see the pool table. "Wow, look at that!" he said as he went over to inspect it.

After a few minutes, the two doors opened and a man wearing khaki slacks and a white button-down shirt entered. He shook my hand and said, "Hello, I'm Nick, nice to meet you."

When he shook my dad's hand, my father asked, "Can we play pool?"

"Sure you can play if you'd like," Nick responded politely, then sat down in one of the chairs.

I started to explain our situation. "We are here because we are looking to see what options we have for my dad to qualify for Medicaid nursing home care."

"I will need to know about any property you own, what balance you have in your checking and savings accounts, what your monthly income is, and any other assets, such as life insurance policies."

"They currently have a business property they own, the house they had in Panama City, and another plot of land has been sold," I replied.

"Okay, how much do you think the business property is worth?" Nick inquired.

"The property appraiser website says it's worth around $400,000, but he co-owns it with his brother, so it would only be half of that," I responded. "They also have a life insurance policy and some burial plots that may be considered assets."

"Yes, the life insurance would be considered an asset," Nick said. "Whose name is on the life insurance policy?"

"It's all in my dad's name." My father had always put everything in his name: the house, the cars, any life insurance or other policies.

Nick then discussed my dad's possible options with us. The eligibility requirements I will list here are only for Florida, as the requirements are different based on what state you reside in.

"For David to be eligible for Medicaid he must not have more than $2,250 in incoming money per month, have an asset limit of $2,000, for instance, in his bank account, and Renee can't have more than a $120,900 asset limit. Assets include properties you own as well."

My parents had already sold two of the three properties they owned; they had a plot of land in Red Bull Island they sold in November 2015, and they had sold their old house in Panama City in January 2016. The only property that remained was the business property that my dad and his brother, Mark, shared.

"The business property will need to be sold and liquidated before we can do the application for David," Nick said to me. "The first thing I recommend we do is get updated powers of attorney to include you and your husband in addition to Renee. I can draw up that paperwork for you to sign in the office on the next visit. The next thing you need to do is get everything transferred into Renee's name: all policies, bank accounts, car titles, and anything else you can think of. Once his name is off the bank account, he will meet the $2,000 saving limit, because he will have no account and he already is under the $2,250 threshold for incoming money per month.

"Once the accounts have all been transferred to Renee's name and the business property is sold, there are three options to get him qualified. The first option is for any amount of money Renee has in the bank account over the $120,900 limit to be put into Medicaid bonds under her name. That means if she had $150,000, to get down to the $120,900 threshold, she would put $29,100 into Medicaid bonds. These bonds have term years that you must keep them in the bond before cashing them out. They also have caveats. For example, if Renee passed away before the term was up on the bond, her estate would lose the money, and the money in the bond would go to Medicaid." This was an option, but it was a risky one.

"The second option is to spend the money over the $120,900 limit," said Nick, but doing this was not desirable either, since my mother was living off the savings.

"The third option is spousal refusal," Nick said. "The spouse refuses to pay for the nursing home care of the other spouse. Choosing this option means Renee would lose all access to your father's incoming money, and his money would be used to pay for the nursing home and his other bills, like life insurance, health insurance, and Medicare health supplement. This option does have a risk, as the state of Florida could sue the refusing spouse for the money that was paid for the nursing care, though being sued for this is a low probability since it has not happened yet to anyone."

We decided to go with spousal refusal and agreed to make a follow-up appointment once we had gotten all the accounts transferred to my mom's name.

During the appointment my dad didn't say much. I don't think he understood what we were talking about. He would perk up and ask questions when we were discussing the business property, but otherwise he didn't seem interested. The only thing that interested him was the pool table. I am sure it reminded him of all his pool playing when he was younger.

My mother removed my dad's name from their checking account and began the process of removing his name from the other policies, too: the business property, my father's life insurance policy, she even had to transfer her name to the title of her own car. It was still in my dad's name even though he hadn't driven for years.

Chapter Eight

More Health Issues

In 2017, we began to notice my dad's feet were swelling. The doctor said he was retaining water, so they put him on a pill to help shed the liquid. The medication, in turn, made him have to urinate a lot. By this point, he could no longer use the bathroom by himself and had to be helped with every step. This entailed leading him to the bathroom, getting him close enough to the toilet, pulling his pants and pull-up down, then telling him to urinate into the toilet, helping put his pants and pull-up back on, washing his hands, and then leading him out of the bathroom back to wherever he had been. He needed assistance with pretty much everything else, too: dressing, brushing his teeth, and directing him on where he needed to go and what he needed to do. He could still, however, feed himself, if the food was prepared for him.

My kids and I would come over and visit my parents on the weekends when I was off. The kids had a playroom at my parents' house, so we'd mainly hang out in there while the kids were playing.

My mom had let me know my dad was falling asleep a lot during the day. We weren't sure what was going on, if it was a sleep problem or a health problem. While we were visiting one Sunday, my dad was out on the couch watching TV and fell asleep sitting up.

I tried to wake him. "Dad, wake up." I pushed his shoulder gently to nudge him. He briefly opened his eyes and went right back to sleep. I nudged him a couple more times, saying, "Dad, wake up are you okay?" That time he did finally wake up all the way.

The next week he was out with the caregiver, Rodney, at the bowling alley. Rodney brought my dad home early and told my mom he was complaining about being too tired to go bowl and about having chest pain. Rodney suggested my mom take him to the ER to get him checked out, which she did.

I got a call later that afternoon from my mom. "I need you to come up to the hospital. Your dad has a blockage in his heart that is causing the episodes of falling asleep. They are saying he is not getting enough blood to his brain. They are doing a procedure to put a splint in his heart."

I rushed to the hospital and spoke with the doctor and my mom. The doctor told us, "With David's Alzheimer's, we believe it would be best to insert a stent while he is under twilight amnesia and awake instead of doing full-blown corrective surgery. Doing surgery would take months of recovery and having anesthetic may set him back even further. I believe inserting the stent in his heart will be the best option for him."

The procedure was to take about an hour according to the doctor. The doctor did not return in an hour; he returned in two hours.

"Everything went well, the stent is in place and working," he said. "It did, however, take a little longer to place it because David was awake, and he kept trying to get up out of the bed while we were placing the stent. The nurse had her hands full trying to keep him in the bed."

Not only had my dad been under the twilight anesthetic, he didn't understand or remember he needed to lie down while they place the splint in his heart. I can only imagine the poor nurse trying to keep him down while they were doing the procedure.

After the stent was inserted, he didn't have any more falling asleep episodes, though, and we were grateful that the heart stent fixed the problem. He had follow-up appointments set to recheck the heart splint and both the leg stents as well as his blood work.

The blood work showed he had diabetes. They prescribed Metformin for him to take. We were instructed to check his blood sugar with a meter twice a day, but he refused to let my mother check it. He complained that the finger prick hurt and that my mother was being mean to him. He did let the nurse check his blood sugar at the doctor's office, but he still complained it hurt.

In May 2017, he had to get another stent placed in his left leg due to another blockage.

All the while, my father's Alzheimer's continued to decline, and he was able to do fewer things. My mother would call me to complain about it, as she had no other outlet. We would speak every day on the phone as we always had, and she would let me know what had happened that morning. It was usually the morning that was the worst.

At night, my father would wake to use the bathroom and could not find it, which sometimes resulted in his urinating on the floor, though usually he would make it to the toilet and urinate on the rug beneath it. My mother and I purchased several cheap bathmats that we could swap out whenever he urinated on them. There were a few occurrences of him not even going to the right room. Sometimes he went to the guestroom and urinated straight onto the carpet. Often, he would step on the urine on the rug and track it back to the couch through the living room.

He would also sometimes try to poop in the middle of the night. He would get that all over the floor and step in it and track it on the floor. Luckily, he insisted on wearing shoes at night, so we put him in tennis shoes that were anti-slip. At this point, my mother had to clean either urine or poop or both every day. It's amazing she didn't go insane.

Occasionally Dad would go in his diaper, and it would leak. That was a whole other story, because my mother had to clean up wherever he was sitting, and get him out of the dirty clothes. If the clothing was too soiled, we would just throw them away. To get him clean, we would put him in the shower to bathe, then get him into fresh, clean clothes. This was when we realized he needed to have twenty-four-hour care.

Chapter Nine

My Time with My Dad

On June 16, 2017, I had just arrived at work and sat down at my desk after dropping off the kids at daycare when I got a call from my mother, and I wasn't able to answer it in time.

Then I got a text saying, "Call me ASAP."

I called back immediately, and my mother told me, "I've slipped and fallen in the bathroom and I can't get up. I think I've broken something. I went into the bathroom in the morning to check if there was urine on the floor and I forgot to wear my non-slip shoes. I didn't see the urine on the floor, and I slipped and fell directly on my knee. It took me about thirty minutes to get your father to bring me my phone so that I could call you."

I immediately talked to my supervisor, got permission to leave work, and went to my parents' house. When I arrived, my mom was on the floor. I tried to get her up, but I couldn't lift her. I told her we'd have to call an ambulance to take her to the hospital.

We had Dad's caregiver coming for his regular weekly visit at 10 a.m. Rodney was not available anymore—he had quit due to some family issues—so another caregiver was scheduled to come. By the time the ambulance got there, the caregiver had also arrived so the paramedics could take my mother to the hospital. As soon as I got the caregiver situated, I followed the ambulance.

"I am going to go to the hospital while they check my mom out," I explained before I left. "Please stay here with my dad, and don't take him anywhere. I will return before you are scheduled to leave at 2p.m."

The caretaker nodded. "Okay, let me know if you need me to do anything else."

When I arrived at the hospital, they already had my mom in one of the rooms, and later gave her an x-ray.

"Her knee is broken in three parts, but it can be fixed surgically and wired back together," the doctor explained. "She doesn't need the surgery today, so we are sending her home and fitting her with an immobilizing brace to wear so that she doesn't bend her knee. I am sending her home with a walker, which she will not be able to walk without, and she needs to minimize how much walking she does."

While we were still at the hospital, the caregiver called to check up. "Your dad is upset and worried, he just wanted to know if she was okay."

"Yes, she is okay. We just found out her knee is broken and we will be back shortly," I replied.

I got my mother's prescriptions, and we were able to get back before the caregiver had to leave. The caregiver helped me get my mother into the house and into bed.

As my mother did absolutely everything for my dad and was now down for the count, I immediately assumed the responsibilities of taking care of both of them. I stayed that night until around 8 p.m. and put them to bed. I was back the next morning around 7 a.m., as my father got up early. My mom closed her door at night because my father would come wandering in looking for her and wake her up multiple times. At this point in his Alzheimer's, he didn't realize the door was shut, and she was in there, so I entered the house and found him wandering around.

"Dad, what are you doing?" I said.

"Just looking around, where is your mother?"

"She's asleep in the bedroom. Let me get you some tea," I said.

I poured some sugar-free tea into his large, red, insulated cup with a straw and went to check on my mother. She was still asleep and not surprisingly had slept badly, but she said the pain meds did help. I helped her get up so she could use the toilet, then helped her to the breakfast table and began making their breakfast. My mother said my dad would need to eat eggs because that's what he liked for breakfast: eggs and fruit. I got the bowl of fruit ready and started frying the eggs. I called my dad to come to the breakfast table.

"Dad, your fruit is ready," I said. I went over to him, he got up, and I took him by the arm and guided him to the breakfast table. Once he sat down in the chair, I found that he no longer knew how to scoot up to the table, so I moved the table to him so he could eat. I went back and got his tea and put it on the table while he began to eat his fruit. For my mother's breakfast, I cut up a grapefruit and gave her half and brought her some water. By then, I realized the eggs were burning.

"Oh crap, the eggs!" I had to make another batch and watch them this time.

While my parents were eating breakfast, I went to check the bathroom rugs. They were soaked with urine, as was part of the bathroom floor. I sprayed bleach on the floor and mopped, then I surveyed the floor to see if there was any tracking of urine onto the hard wood. There was, so I mopped that area with some vinegar and water, then followed by mopping with alcohol. Once the bathroom floor was dried, I put out clean rugs and put the urine-soaked rugs in the washing machine. I did a few other things around the house for the animals, fed the cats and dogs, cleaned the cat boxes, and vacuumed up the cat litter that was on the floor. My mother had a very old cat with a litter box in the bathroom near the shower, and it irritated my father if there was cat litter on the floor.

Once my parents finished breakfast, it was time to give them their morning medications. I went and got my mother's pill holder and gave it to her, then I got my father's medications ready to give to him. He had around seven pills he needed to take in the morning, ranging from smaller to larger capsules. He didn't like to take them, and he had a tough time swallowing the bigger capsules.

"Okay, Dad, time to take your medicine," I said. I refilled his drink. He sometimes had to drink two thirty-two-ounce cups of tea to get everything down since he had such a hard time swallowing. Occasionally, he would hide the pills or spit them out. My mother often found pills on the floor, and we were so thankful that the kids, cats, and dogs didn't see them and eat them.

"These aren't my pills, I don't need them," my dad responded.

"Yes, they are your pills, and the doctor prescribed them for you. Look, Mom is taking her pills the doctor prescribed for her. Can you take them for me?"

He responded reluctantly. "Yes."

I gave him the first pill, starting out with a smaller one. I put it in his hand and said, "Okay, put the pill in your mouth, then drink some tea and swallow it."

It took me repeating the instructions a few times, but finally he did it. We continued on, but when we got the capsules, it was difficult for him to swallow them. I felt really bad for him; I could see him struggling to swallow and taking more sips of the tea. I was honestly afraid sometimes that he was going to choke on the capsules.

It was always hit-and-miss for him taking the medicines. Some days he would take them fine, other days he would resist, and sometimes we would have to repeat the instructions over and over again. Occasionally, my mother would get annoyed and raise her voice. I told her to try not to do that, no matter how frustrating it was, because it aggravated my dad and then he would not do what we were asking. When I was giving him his medications, I would calmly repeat the same instructions until he finally did it. Very soon he got to the point to where he wouldn't take the pills at all, and my mother had to use a pill crusher and give them to him in ice cream. He liked sweets, so it was a good way to get him to take his medication without him knowing.

Once we were done with the morning medications, it was time for him to take a shower. He liked to take a shower in the mornings. I laid out his clothes: pants, shirt, undershirt, and pull-up diaper. I started the water in the shower—he liked it hot before he got in. Then I led him into the bedroom so I could sit him on the bed to undress him. I took his clothes off then led him to the bathroom so he could get in the shower. We had a safety handrail installed on the wall inside the shower. I told him to hold onto it as he stepped into the shower. He seemed confused at first, but once I repeated it, he got into the shower while holding the bar. I handed him his rag, and he got his soap and started to wash. He was still able to do that. He did, however, need help to wash his hair, and he was usually not cooperative for that.

While he was in the shower, I put his dirty clothes in the hamper and went to talk to my mother. "I didn't realize he was this bad; he needs help with most everything."

"Yes." She nodded. I think she had tried to shield me from how bad it was, and that was sweet of her.

After about ten minutes, my dad turned off the water in the shower, which meant he was ready to get out. I grabbed the towel and went to the shower, opened it, and told him to step out onto the rug. We had a series of rugs for him to walk over from the shower to the bedroom carpet. I dried him off, led him to the bed, and instructed him to sit down. I got him dressed, putting his pull-up on first, followed by his undershirt, then shirt, pants, socks, and shoes. He usually had a hard time with the shirt, he would forget he needed to put his arm back to get it into the sleeve. Once he was dressed, I led him back to the living room so he could sit on the couch. I put on one of his favorite movies, *No Time for Sergeants*. I watched the whole movie with him. I had never seen it before. It was actually pretty funny, and he really enjoyed it.

He needed to use the bathroom, so I led him to the bathroom, helped him pull his pants down, and told him to aim for the toilet. Most of the time he was able to urinate in the toilet, but sometimes he missed. After he was done, I helped him get his pants back up, pointed to the sink, and told him to wash his hands while I turned the water on. I put soap on his hands. He immediately started washing his hands—that was one thing he still excelled at. I handed him the paper towel to dry his hands, then threw it in the trash for him as he usually just looked around searching for a trash can to throw it away in, then led him back to the couch.

After one particular incident, I was careful to observe him while he was washing his hands. One weekend when I was watching my parents and my two small children, my son told me he needed a new diaper, and that distracted me. I had just helped my dad use the bathroom and told my dad to wash his hands and pointed at the sink. I left momentarily to check my son's diaper. When I came back, my dad was washing his hands in the toilet. Luckily, the toilet had already been flushed. My mom noticed at the same time I did and redirected him to use the sink.

By this point, it was almost time for lunch. I prepared my parents' meal and served it to them. After that, we watched the same movie a few more times. Then I prepped their food for dinner. I served them dinner and then got my dad to take his nighttime pills, and left to go home to my family and children. I was fortunate that my husband was able to watch my children and care for them while I was with my parents.

My continual care for them went on for about a week and a half until I could find a caretaker service to come and stay with them during the day, so I could go back to work. I finally found a caretaker service that could do what we needed, and they started coming Monday through Friday. I would continue to care for my parents on Saturday and Sundays.

My mother had a follow-up appointment the next week. At the appointment, the doctor scheduled her for surgery to repair her knee and took pre-op blood work and an EKG. The caregiver watched my dad while I took her to the appointment.

After my mother's knee surgery, she was in a lot of pain and had to use a wheelchair. At her six-week follow-up appointment, the doctor said she could use a walker and get up and walk around a bit. My mother was overjoyed that she could finally start getting around. She is the type of person that likes to be constantly doing things, such as taking care of my dad, and was happy to be getting back to that.

<div align="center">~~~</div>

As my father progressed, his hallucinations gradually became less benign. He had a few items that he loved to carry around in a small, rectangular cedar box he had got when he was a boy. It was made by Marston & Quina downtown, and we think one of his grandparents gave it to him. He liked to keep a few things of his things in there, a few poker chips, an old watch, and some coins from his collection. He would take the items out, look at them, and leave them out on the table without putting them back in the box. My mother would put the items back in the box when she was straightening up.

One Sunday morning I came over to find my dad wandering around the house. He came up to me, fuming, and said, "She is a thief and stole my stuff!"

"Who is a thief? Do you mean Mom?" I replied.

"She's a thief!" he repeated angrily.

He had a bizarre expression on his face. He was generally happy and smiling unless he was agitated. This time, since his hallucination wasn't benign, I tried to reason with him.

"Dad, Mom is not a thief," I said. "She was probably just cleaning up your stuff."

I took him over to the box and showed him the items were there, which seemed to help. Then I went and woke up my mom, and she came out. My father's body language still was a bit hostile towards her, but I redirected him to his fruit bowl, which was waiting for him at the breakfast table, and he seemed to forget all about it.

My mother told me the day before he had had a similar outburst while the caregiver was there. It went on for about an hour before they got him to snap out of it.

After breakfast, I got his pills and said, "Take the pill and put it in your mouth and then take some tea and swallow it." He started crying, so I asked him, "What's wrong?"

He told me sadly, "I used to be able to do all these things, and now I can't."

"It's okay, Dad, I'm here to help you," I told him. I felt so sad because this showed he did have some moments of clarity and he realized that he couldn't do a lot of the things he used to and he was upset about it. Alzheimer's is a cruel disease.

Chapter Ten

My Mother's Recovery

As my mother recovered from her knee surgery, my father continued to decline. He had more episodes of agitation and his hostility was directed toward my mother. We think it may have had to do with so many different people coming into the house. The caregiver sent by the company we were using was not always the same one, and there were several nurses and physical and occupational therapists from home health care that would come over.

My mother called me to tell me about one episode in particular. I was on the way home from work.

"Hey, it's me, I wanted to tell you about what your father did today," she said.

"What happened?" I asked in a worried voice.

"I was in the bedroom with the caregiver and your father. We were getting him ready to take his shower. He started yelling loudly, 'I WANT EVERYONE OUT OF THE HOUSE NOW!' Then he said he was going to start kicking us," she said in a scared voice. My mother had started to feel unsafe: my father was bigger than her, and even though he was unsteady, if he had hit her or kicked her it could have hurt.

"We need to start looking for a nursing home for him," I said. "He is having more agitated and hostile episodes." I was becoming worried about my father's increasing anger towards my mother. He had never acted on it and hurt her physically, but I was worried that in the future he might. I made an appointment with our elder law attorney, Nick, and arranged for a caregiver to watch my dad this time while we went to the appointment.

~~~

Nick came into the meeting room. "Good afternoon, it's good to see you again."

We started to discuss that we wanted to look for a nursing home for my dad. "Now that the business property is sold, what else do we need to do to be ready to apply for Medicaid?" I asked.
~~~

Nick reviewed the policies with us and talked about what was still in my father's name and what assets they had. "The only thing you still need to get moved into your mother's name is the life insurance policy. When that is done and you've located a nursing home, we can go ahead and start the Medicaid application."

While my mother contacted the life insurance company to get the policy changed to her name from my dad's, I began looking for nursing homes. I had no idea where to start, so I turned to the Internet to research them. I started looking for homes located close to us. I called several of them and asked if they accepted Medicaid, and if so, did they have any rooms and could we do a tour.

I found an assisted living facility that was close to our house. At that time, I didn't realize that Medicaid would only pay in full for nursing homes and not assisted living facilities. My dad went with us. He didn't seem to understand why we were touring the place or that it was an assisted living facility. He just enjoyed going as an outing and getting to look around. I was not impressed with the facility: all the floors were concrete and the Medicaid rooms were tiny and had two beds each. Worst of all, they had a bathroom that was shared with the room right next to them, which meant four people using one bathroom. That would definitely not work with my father having accidents on the floor. We continued the tour and entered the activities room where all the residents were playing bingo.

"Hello, everybody!" said my dad in a loud voice as he walked in. He immediately began trying to engage the residents in conversation. I had to lead him out of the room after a while, as he wanted to stay and talk to more of the residents.

We toured a few more nursing homes. Some were very nice but had a very long waiting list (one list was up to five years), and some we didn't like. When I was calling around to different nursing homes, one of them said that if we had home health care services, we could ask the home health care social worker to send out packets to see if there were any Medicaid rooms available. They referred to the Medicaid rooms as "Medicaid beds." I was significantly relieved as there was finally someone that could help me search for somewhere for my dad. I spoke to the social worker at our home health care agency, and she began searching for availability. This went on for around one and a half months, but nothing in Pensacola was available.

<center>~~~</center>

Because of this, my mom decided to activate hospice care. I did not know this before, but hospice care can be activated even though the patient is not at the end of life stage. My mother did it so she could get help with my dad. Though they did have caregivers coming, my dad frequently refused to let them bathe or dress him, so my mother was still doing this even in her healing state. When she activated the hospice care, they came three times a week and would help with bathing, dressing, and trimming my dad's beard. Most days, he allowed them to help care for him. For some reason he would not let my mother shave his beard or shampoo his hair, but the hospice nurses were able to help with that.

My mother also contacted the hospice social worker to see if she might have more luck finding my dad a Medicaid bed than the home health care social worker. It took a few weeks to get my dad's paperwork transferred from the home health care social worker, but once it was I quickly received a call from the hospice social worker.

"Hi, this is Jane with Emerald Coast Hospice, I am the social worker assigned to your dad's case. I have found a private Medicaid bed for your father," she said.

I responded with excitement. "That's great! Where is it, and what does 'private' mean?" Medicaid beds usually had two residents per room, so I figured private probably meant one resident.

"It's at Bayside, and it means that it only has one bed in the room. You will have to pay an extra four hundred and sixty-five dollars a month in addition to what Medicaid pays."

"Okay, that's not too bad," I responded. "Let me call and talk to my mother about it and see what she thinks."

We hung up, and I immediately called my mother to discuss the opening at Bayside. Once I explained everything, she agreed to go on a tour. I called the nursing home and set up a tour for that Friday. I also called Nick to let him know what was going on and texted the social worker to let her know our plans.

My parents met me at the nursing home to do the tour. It was in a nice area of town, near the bluffs and bay. The home was in a white, two-story building with two parking lots and a drive-through where you could drop off your loved one at the front door. My mom and dad used an Uber to get there. I arrived at the same time, parked, and went to help my mom get my dad out of the taxi in the drive-through.

As we entered the building, a woman headed towards us. She was in her mid-thirties, had shoulder-length brown hair, and smiled as she met us at the door.

"Hello, you must be April, Renee, and David. I'm Molly, the head of the business office, I'll be giving the tour," she said continuing to smile.

"Hello, nice to meet you. Thank you for giving us a tour on such short notice," I said.

"Oh, 'course, no problem at all. Right this way! We will start on the first floor..." The first floor was for rehabilitation services. They had a common room, and the residents were playing bingo as we passed by. The residents looked like they were enjoying the game. This floor had an outdoor area that was fenced in so that the residents could go outside.

"They do outside movies once a week in the outdoor area," Molly said as we walked through it.

"Oh, that's cool," I said.

"Now we will head up to the second floor. That's where we have the long-term care rooms and the available private Medicaid room," she said.

We took the elevator up, and she led us down the hall to the room. It did not smell of urine like some of the other nursing homes we had toured, and the room was near the nurse's station, so that was a plus. It had white vinyl floors, a private bathroom with a toilet, sink, and walk-in tile shower, and a twin bed with a gold pleated bedspread, small flat-screen TV, two chairs, and a dark wood nightstand. The two windows, which looked out on the rooftop, did not open and appeared green from the inside.

We found the room acceptable, so we went to discuss reserving it for my dad.

"We'd like to take the room; we are working with Nick on the Medicaid application," I said.

Molly nodded. "Yes, we have worked with him on Medicaid applications for residents here before. I will have the financial office reach out to him. Once they have the arrangements for the financial part squared away, he can move in."

I was very relieved at that point, as we had finally found somewhere for my dad to live. Even though we'd have to pay the extra money every month due to the room being private, I thought it was the best thing for my father. He didn't like a lot of noise and activity, which could agitate him, so once he moved in, he eventually started eating in his room because the cafeteria was too loud for him. It was nice when we were visiting with him and could have the privacy as well.

During the tour, we got a wheelchair for my dad since it was a lot of walking and he got tired. He was oblivious to why we were touring, just as he was on the other nursing home tours. He was just happy to be out of the house.

Chapter Eleven

Disco Bowling

My mother was having second thoughts about letting my dad move into the nursing home. She was at her limit and no longer able to care for him but still felt terrible about moving him in. Unlike her, I knew it was what needed to be done and I didn't have regrets—that is, until we moved him in.

I got the call the week after our tour: Bayside had the financial part worked out. Nick was applying for Medicaid for my dad, and they had authorized my dad to go ahead and move in on Friday, November 3. Once the application was approved, Medicaid would pay retroactively to the date my dad moved in.

Over the next few days, my mother got my father's things ready to go to the nursing home. She packed his pants, shirts, undershirts, socks, pajama pants, and pull-ups. They said we could bring a DVD player and a few DVDs, as well as some personal effects, but were advised not to bring anything too expensive "as things can go missing." Either my father could misplace it, or one of the other residents might mistake it for theirs and take it. There were a substantial number of Alzheimer's patients on the second floor with him.

My mother packed two of his favorite blankets (a fleece blanket with a deer on it and a red one), a picture of his grandparents, a picture of my mom and dad together, and his favorite cedar chest box with a few of his poker chips, a deck of cards, and pretend money.

I took time off work the day we moved him in so that I could take him and my mother up there. When I arrived at my parents' house, my mom quietly gave me the things to pack into the car. We didn't want to alert him to what was going on because we were worried he would get agitated, wouldn't get into the car, and might fight us.

I felt pretty guilty doing this, but we didn't tell him beforehand where we were going or that he was moving into the nursing home. I am not sure that if we had told him he would have understood. We arrived at Bayside at 10 a.m., and we took him in first before bringing his things up. The nurse was waiting for us in the lobby with a wheelchair for my dad and escorted us upstairs. In his room, my dad got out of the wheelchair and sat on the bed.

"This bed is comfortable," he said as he lay down on it.

I got a cart and went downstairs to get the rest of his stuff. It took two trips to fetch everything. Once I got everything upstairs, the business operations head, Molly, was talking to my mom and getting her to sign a few things. I unpacked my dad's clothes and put them in the closet, put his toiletries in the bathroom, and attempted to hook up the DVD player. There was an issue with the TV not working, so the nurse had to call maintenance to fix the TV.

My mom and I decided we were going to stay for a while and eat lunch with my dad. Lunch was served at noon, so we headed down the cafeteria around 11:45 and found a table to sit at. We asked one of the nurses whether we served ourselves, and she told us they would bring lunch to us at the table. They brought all three of us our meals at once: fried fish, coleslaw, cheese grits, and canned fruit salad. The food was actually good. I was impressed!

My dad was pleased, too. "This place is great, they bring the food to you and it's good!" he said. He seemed happy being there.

After lunch, I looked at the bulletin board in his room with the listed activities for the residents: today's activity after lunch was twilight bowling. Bowling was the perfect activity for my dad.

"They have twilight bowling in a few minutes, do you want to go?" I asked my dad.

"Yes!" he said excitedly.

I went and talked to the activities coordinator, Kate, and she told me they'd be doing the bowling in the cafeteria. We went down to the cafeteria right before it was time for the bowling to start and Kate was setting up the bowling pins. They used real bowling pins, but for the ball, they used a children's bouncy ball. She let my dad go first and bowl. He was having a great time.

Kate helped instruct him on throwing the ball to hit the pins, then walked over to my mother and me. She was short, with blond hair and plastic-rimmed glasses. We told her we were going to leave soon and asked how we should approach that.

"Alzheimer's patients live in the now, so it's better if you leave without saying goodbye," she told us. "This way it will be less upsetting to him."

My mother and I didn't want to do that as we felt extremely guilty for leaving him there in the first place with strangers, let alone without saying goodbye.

"What will you say when he starts asking about my mom or me?" I asked.

"We tell them you went to work or you're out shopping, and you'll be back later," she said.

"Okay, should we come back tomorrow?" I asked.

"It's probably better to stay away a few days so he can acclimate," Kate responded.

"Would Monday be okay then?"

"Yes," she said.

"Okay, we will head out then."

Kate went back over to help my dad, and we left the cafeteria. We went to my dad's room to get some of the boxes we were going to take back home with us. Once we got into the room, my mother broke down.

"I can't do this, I can't leave him here!" she said.

"I know, I don't want to either, but we need to," I told her. "It's best for him and he will be able to get around-the-clock care here."

We left and went to the car. I dropped off my mother at her house and then headed home to mine. After I got back, I started to feel really guilty. I felt so horrible for leaving him there and not even saying goodbye! I worried about whether he would be okay there, whether he would be treated well, and if he would continue to eat properly. He always ate so well at home, but we made him whatever he wanted.

The nurse told us we could call the second-floor nurse's station anytime and check on my dad, so my mom called a few hours after we had dropped him off. My mom and I were anxious that he would freak out once he realized we weren't there. To the contrary, the nurse said once he realized we weren't there, he asked, "Where are my wife and daughter?"

The nurse told him, "They are out shopping and will be back later."

"Okay," he said, and went on without issue. I was so happy to hear he didn't get upset, as that was something I had been very concerned about.

The next morning my mom called again to check and see how he was. The nurse reported that he hadn't slept that night but otherwise was doing okay, and that he had only asked about us once. We found out later they had only given him one instead of the two sleeping pills he usually got so perhaps that was why.

On Monday my mom went to visit him, and he was pleased to see her. He immediately complained. "I don't like the people here and want to go home."

He did that in the beginning when we visited him, complaining that he didn't like the people there and that they were mean. It was hard to tell if he didn't like them, or maybe it was because it wasn't us taking care of him.

I still felt terrible hearing him say this. I knew it was best for him, but I still worried.

The nurse called my mother the next day. My dad was wandering all over the place and went to one of the female resident's rooms, tried to sit on the bed, and fell off. He was okay and uninjured, but the nursing home had decided to give him a one-on-one aide to stay with him, since he was ambulatory and wandering around. It upset some of the female residents having a male come into their room, so the one-on-one was there both to keep him from doing that and to help him with whatever task he was doing. I was delighted they offered this service, and that it wasn't any extra cost for the one-on-one aide. Dad needed twenty-four-hour supervision, and when he was home either my mom or I were with him at all times except when he was sleeping. At home, the doctor had prescribed some sleeping pills so my dad would sleep at night. A few times, he had gone outside at night while my mother was sleeping and wandered around the neighborhood. Fortunately, those times he still remembered how to get back to the house. On one of the occurrences, he told us the next day he had gone outside and saw some orange intestines out in the yard. What he saw were orange drainage pipes the city had stored in the lot next to their house. Another time my mother was awakened to a beeping sound outside. My father was in the backyard with his metal detector. She never found out what exactly he was looking for, but he was trying to find something.

At first he wasn't very cooperative with the one-on-one. He didn't want to follow directions or let the nurses help him change his diaper. After being there for two weeks, he didn't use the toilet anymore—he only went in his diaper. He gave the hospice nurses a hard time when they tried to bathe him.

We (and the nursing home) realized a few weeks after he moved in that my dad did not like the women nurses telling him what to do, so Bayside hired a male one-on-one specifically for my father. His name was James, and he was a tall, big-boned young man with short, braided hair. He was very kind to my father, kinder than any of the other one-on-ones he had had, and he looked for ways to try and find different activities that my dad enjoyed.

I would take the kids up on the weekend to see their grandpa, and my mom would go with us. One week, we saw James bringing my dad back from being outside in the first floor outdoor area.

"Hello, we were outside," he said. "I just wanted to try something different for David and see if he liked it."

My dad didn't like it that day because it was chilly outside and he got cold easily. During our last visit, we had brought in some pictures we had taken for Christmas with the kids, but had forgotten to bring push-pins so we could put them on his bulletin board. When we arrived in the room this time, I realized James had taken the pictures, lined them up perfectly, and stapled them to the bulletin board for us! I was so pleasantly surprised; my dad loved looking at the pictures of the kids on the bulletin board. It was very sweet of James to take it upon himself to do that. I think he genuinely enjoyed being there with my dad and helping him.

After the first few weeks, my dad stopped saying he wanted to go home and said to my mother, "Can I come with you to your house?" He seemed to be acclimating to being in the nursing home and forgetting about their old house. But over the next few weeks, we noticed he had lost a lot of weight.

~~~

We had our first care meeting in December right before Christmas, which was an appointment with the social worker for the nursing home, the head nurse, and the hospice folks to discuss how my dad was doing and any plans we wanted or needed. My mother and I arrived and headed into the office downstairs for the meeting. Two of the nurses from hospice were already there, Beth and Julie, both in their blue scrubs, so we sat down at the table and waited for Ruth, the head nurse on the second floor, and Donald, the social worker.

Donald and Ruth arrived a few minutes later, and we started the meeting.

"I am concerned with the amount of weight my father has lost while being here. After only eight weeks, he looks visibly thinner," I began.

Ruth responded while looking at her notes. "Yes, looking at our records he was two hundred eleven pounds when he entered, and at his last weigh-in it's showing he is one hundred and eighty pounds."

When he entered the nursing home, he was slightly overweight, and the swelling in his feet from the water was contributing to that.

"He hasn't been eating well at every meal either," she continued. "He doesn't like what they have on the menu for the day, so we will order off the special menu for him, usually an egg salad sandwich." My father loved egg salad, and my mother and I had made it a lot for him at home. He ate it for breakfast, lunch, and sometimes even dinner, though he preferred ham or egg sandwiches or hot dogs for dinner with a small salad. For snacks, we would cut up plenty of fresh fruit—watermelon, grapes or strawberries. They didn't have fresh fruit on the menu, but at least they had his egg salad sandwiches.

Before entering the nursing home, my father had complained about a tooth bothering him. My mother had taken him to their dentist, but he refused to open his mouth. We thought maybe the tooth was hurting him
~~~

and that was what was preventing him from eating. Bayside had a dentist that came on site and visited the patients, but it seemed he had had similar problems.

"Yes, he did come last month, but your father would not open his mouth for the dentist," Ruth said.

"Maybe they could give him a sedative to help him relax before the dentist got there?" I asked, as I turned to look at the hospice nurses.

Hospice was in charge of all of my father's medications. In turn, they were his doctors now, prescribing and changing medication as needed. Bayside would then administer the medication hospice prescribed to my father.

"Yes, we can give him something to calm him before the dentist arrives," Julie said.

"I will come up here, too, to help tell him he has to let the dentist examine him. Just let me know what time it is scheduled," said my mother.

"I will let you know as soon as we get the schedule," Ruth responded.

"Okay, thanks," I said. "Next, I'd like to discuss his medications. My mother has told me my father has been taken off some pills: the blood pressure tablets and Namzaric, the Alzheimer's medication."

Julie confirmed this was correct, and that because of his weight loss his blood pressure had dropped to a normal level.

"Okay, well, that's a good thing," I replied. "Why was the Namzaric stopped?" I already knew the answer but wanted to hear it from the hospice nurse. The first part was that Namzaric was not a covered medication for Medicare after you had activated hospice. Once hospice is activated, certain medications and procedures are no longer covered, for example, diagnostic procedures such as CAT scans. The separate medications that made up Namzaric—memantine HCl & donepezil HCl— were covered, though, so he could have been switched to those.

"With Alzheimer's patients there comes a time when that medication is no longer effective," responded Julie. "In your father's case, it is no longer helping him slow the progression of the disease."

"I understand," I said. The last time my dad had seen the neurologist before being admitted to the nursing home, the doctor stated that my dad shouldn't be declining into later stages of Alzheimer's as fast as he was on the medication. So maybe the hospice was right about that. I often wonder if taking him off the medication was the right choice, because afterwards things got much worse.

"I have something I'd like to bring up," Ruth said next. "Your father has had some outbursts at the nursing home. One of the female nurses was trying to wake him up last week, and he grabbed her braided hair and began pulling it."

"I'm so sorry, he's never done anything like that at home!" I said.

"He also slugged one nurse in the face, but she said that he was startled and she believes that's why it happened. He hit another nurse with the golf club."

"Oh my God, you're not serious?" I asked, shocked. Both my mother and I were stunned, mortified, and embarrassed at the same time. My father had made threats before, but he had never actually got physical. We had taken the golf club and putting green up there for him to use since he wasn't interested in the other activities they were doing.

"Do you want us to take the golf club home?" I asked.

"Yes, that would be a good idea. But he's okay unless he gets agitated or something triggers him," Ruth said.

We adjourned the meeting and headed up to see my dad. My mother distracted him while I took the golf club out of the closet so we could take it with us.

My father had threatened my mother when he was still at home, but it had never gotten to a physical confrontation. I wonder now if it could have escalated to that point if we hadn't admitted him at the time we did.

~~~

Each Saturday when we visited with my children, my father was happy to see us, especially the kids. His eyes always lit up when he saw Eva and Diego, and he smiled. He loved the grandchildren more than anything.

But over the next few weeks, when we talked to him, he would start saying gibberish that didn't make sense. He would say things that didn't belong together. For instance, one day he told me, "We need to... the fence, can you get that for me?" I told him that, yes, I would take care of it for him. Based on his reaction, my response put him at ease. He thought I understood what he meant. It was getting harder for him to communicate effectively with the outside world.

We visited the Saturday before Christmas to bring him his presents. My great-uncle Abe, great-aunt Bobbie, great-aunt Joanne, and cousin Shane came to visit him as well.

Uncle Abe was my Grandfather Papaw's younger brother, and he had just had eye surgery to remove cataracts, so his eyes were slightly red. He had always been kind to my family and me, and his wife, Aunt Bobbie, was a beautiful woman even in her seventies. My cousin Shane accompanied them in his thick-rimmed glasses. Aunt Joanne, my grandfather's younger sister, wore glasses, too, as did pretty much all of my grandfather's siblings. Aunt Joanne was very kind to us as well, and always took an interest in the
~~~

things we were doing. I feel like after my grandfather died, she took over "being there" for us.

When we arrived in my father's room, he had pooped in his diaper, and the nurses were trying to clean him up, so we headed to the atrium to wait there for him with the rest of the family. The atrium was the second floor's common room. The walls on the exterior were glass, and you could see into the parking lot. The kids loved being in that room and staring through the glass. After about ten minutes my mother went to check on my father, as he had been giving the nurses a hard time and didn't want to have his diaper changed. Once my mother told him that everyone was waiting and he needed to let the nurse change him, he finally relented and came into the atrium to be with everyone. Uncle Abe, Aunt Bobbie, Aunt Joanne, and Shane went over to see my dad and hug him hello.

"Hey," my father said with a smile. My mother guided him to the couch where she assisted him in sitting down.

"David, we've brought your Christmas presents for you to open!" she said.

My dad said, "Okay," still smiling, though he didn't seem interested.

I got the presents and started bringing them over to him one by one. He just looked at them and didn't seem to know what to do with them.

"Dad, open your present, that's from Mom," I said.

He didn't open the present, so Eva opened it for him. It was a few shirts and pajama pants. He just set them to the side uninterested.

"Okay, Eva, bring Grandpa his next present. This is from me," I said.

Once again, she opened the present for him, and it was the blue Sherpa blanket I had bought him. He put the blanket on his lap and covered his legs.

The last present was from Eva and Diego. Eva opened it, and it was a small bronze pocket watch that said "The Greatest Grandpa." Just as before, he seemed uninterested, and Eva took the pocket watch.

"Eva, bring me the watch so I can put it back in the case for Grandpa. He can look at it later," I said.

Over the next few weeks, my father continued to lose weight, and only about fifty percent of what he said made sense. He started having problems with his balance and was falling over, so hospice ordered a high-backed wheelchair for him. He used the wheelchair to roam the halls instead of walking, and got around very well in it.

In mid-January 2018, we took a family vacation to Disney World, and after we returned we brought my dad a Mickey Mouse hat. It was a red, white, and blue ball cap with a red Mickey on the top, which my mother had picked it out.

"Hi, Dad, we brought you a hat with Mickey Mouse on it," I said.

"Look, David, it's from Disney World," my mother said. She walked over and put the hat on his head.

He responded, "Okay," then said something in gibberish that wasn't even English.

"Eva and Diego, go say hi to Grandpa," I said. Eva went over, and I picked her up so she could sit on his lap. He hugged her, and I snapped a few photos. Diego was next, and I put him on Grandpa's lap, too, and he got a hug as well.

"Hi Grandpa," Diego said, then squirmed out so he could go run around the room. It was often hard to get both of them to stay still when visiting, so we only visited for short amounts of time with the kids.

That was the last time I saw my dad when he was really *there.* He was not making total sense when he talked, but he was interacting with us and the kids in conversation, and he hugged them like he had not seen them in forever.

Over the next three weeks, we were unable to visit my dad. It was February, and the flu had ramped up in our area as well as the whole country. His nursing home had cases of the flu on his floor, and they were on quarantine, so no one could visit. The next week, my dad started running a 102.7 fever. He had never had a fever that high in his life, even when he had pneumonia. He had no other symptoms, but they treated it as flu and gave him Tamiflu medicine. The following week, my son Diego got sick with the flu, too, so we didn't visit my dad so he wouldn't be exposed.

In those three weeks, my father declined severely. On our next visit, I could see that he had lost so much weight that he looked skeletal. His face was so thin that you could see his cheekbones sticking out. When he smiled at us, his jaw was open, and he didn't close his mouth the entire visit. He had stopped using his left arm entirely. Losing the ability to remember how to use your limbs is a part of the disease because, in the later stages, the brain stops sending commands to use the arms and legs. That's why Alzheimer's patients are eventually bedridden and can no longer get up.

The next time we visited, we arrived at lunchtime, and Aunt Joanne was there, too. She said the nurses were struggling to feed my father, who was looking extremely thin. We found him out in the hallway with a tray still full of food over his wheelchair.

"He's only eating about twenty-five percent of his food," one of the nurses confirmed. "We try to feed it to him, but he just won't eat that much."

I went over to my father. "Hi Dad, Eva and Diego are here to see you."

He didn't look up when I spoke, instead staring off at something down the hallway. I picked up Diego and held him in front of my dad, and when he saw his grandson he smiled. He said something, but I couldn't make it out. He was speaking very quietly, mumbling softly. The nurse took my father to his room, and we followed.

While we were in his room, though, my dad did not interact with us. He started rolling toward the pictures on the bulletin board. My mother went over to talk to him and said, "David, how are you doing?" He mumbled something quietly that she couldn't make out.

With the good arm he could still use, he reached out to touch a picture of Diego and Eva on the bulletin board. In the photo, Eva was wearing her white faux-fur jacket with silver sequins, clutching her small blue teddy bear and smiling brightly. Diego, with his shoulder length curly dark brown hair, was seated next to her, wearing his blue button-down shirt with a huge grin. My father continued to reach forward, rolling his wheelchair toward the picture, until he hit the wall. He stopped moving, his eyes were closed, but his mouth was still open. I realized right away he had fallen asleep. We notified the nurse that he was sleeping, as they were now checking on him every fifteen minutes and had removed the one-on-one since he was not as active.

After visiting him, I was pretty upset. I knew it wasn't going to be long before he died at this rate. He was incredibly thin and not eating or drinking much.

My husband didn't usually come with us to visit my dad, but when I got home I told him, "You need to come with us next weekend to see my dad. He is not doing well, and I don't believe it will be long."

"Okay, yes," my husband said. "I want to go with you. I want to see him before he dies."

Chapter Twelve

The End

We planned for my husband to come and visit my father with us the next Saturday, but my mother went to visit him on Monday and called to tell me he wasn't doing well.

"He won't get up out of bed, and they said he has been lethargic since Sunday," she said.

"Has he eaten anything?" I asked.

"No, he hasn't. They are switching him to a pureed diet to see if he will eat. He barely responded to me, but once I got him to look at me he said, 'Pretty,'" she said. I honestly think that's all he could make out at that time. He was trying to communicate with her, and that's the best he could do.

"I talked to the hospice nurse today, she said he is pre-imminent," my mother continued. That is as bad as it sounds: when they classify someone as imminent, that means they will die very soon, and my dad was in the stage right before that. "The hospice nurse told me there is no way to tell how long he will be in this stage."

My heart dropped. My gut feeling that he was going to die seemed to be coming true. I secretly hoped that he'd be able to eat and recover, but I knew that was not a likely scenario.

"The nurse told me she thinks he is losing his ability to swallow, that's why he's not eating or drinking," my mother said. Losing the ability to swallow was even worse news. If he was unable to swallow, he couldn't eat or drink and wouldn't survive.

My mother visited another few times during the week. There was no change. My father was still not eating or drinking, was barely responsive, and would not get out of the bed.

On Saturday, it was my son's third birthday party. My entire family, including my husband, went to visit my dad beforehand. When we arrived, they had him propped up with the bed raised so he was sitting. He was awake and staring blankly at the TV with his mouth open. He was shivering and had taken his good arm out of the white undershirt he was wearing. His socked feet stuck out of the covers. We checked the thermostat, which was set to cold, so we turned it off. I called the nurse and told her we couldn't get his arm back in the shirt, so she came in and took care of it. Then my husband covered my father up with the blanket, and he fell asleep. I tried to wake him a few times, and he would open his eyes, but immediately closed them again. One time in particular, we put Diego in his line of sight so he could see him. He smiled at Diego and that proved to me, even with how far gone he was, that he was still there. He loved both Diego and Eva dearly. My mother put Diego on the bed, and Diego patted him on the head and hugged him goodbye. The rest of us said our goodbyes and hugged him, then left. That was the last time I saw my father smile.

The next morning, I was putting away groceries and starting to load the slow cooker with chicken wings for dinner when I received a call from my mother.

"We need to go to Bayside now. They just called me and said his kidneys are shutting down," my mother said in a trembling voice. "They don't know how long it will be."

"Okay, we will be there in a few minutes to pick you up," I said, feeling as if my heart had been crushed. We hung up, and I immediately went to talk to my husband.

"We need to go now. The nursing home just called, and my father's kidneys are shutting down."

I scrambled to get the kids ready while my husband finished getting ready himself. I put up the food I had in the slow cooker, and then we left to pick up my mother.

When we arrived at the nursing home, we went straight into my father's room. My dad was in bed, and his mouth was still open. It was covered by an oxygen mask. His eyes were half open, too, but they were rolled back in his head. He was not dressed in his regular clothes. Instead he was wearing a blue-and-white polka-dot hospital gown. The nurse came in and immediately brought extra chairs.

"We have been giving him morphine to keep him comfortable, and he is wearing the oxygen mask to help him breathe," she explained. Thankfully, the hospice nurse had ordered the morphine and oxygen tank for him last week in case we had needed it for the weekend. I was glad that she did. I was told that once the organs start to shut down, it is very painful, and the morphine was to keep him from feeling it.

My mother and I went over to talk to my dad, but he was not responsive. He was responsive a couple of times the day before, so I think it was probably the morphine keeping him like that. He was so thin, so the dose they were giving him to keep him comfortable was probably high. The nurse came back a bit later and gave him morphine from a tiny dropper bottle. She placed one drop under his tongue, as she did hourly. She also checked his temperature and said he had been running a fever. There is something called terminal fever, and the hospice nurse explained to us later that when the body is shutting down, there is inflammation that raises the body temperature.

Around thirty minutes later the nurse came in with a tray of food with ham, turkey, and cheese sandwiches, a pitcher of orange juice, a pitcher of water, and some cookies. I thanked her. I was very touched at that moment that they had brought us something from the cafeteria to eat while we were waiting. I felt really grateful for the food. We ate some of the sandwiches, and Diego had the cheese while Eva helped herself to some of the turkey meat.

By that time, Aunt Joanne had arrived to wait with us. She was on her way to church, and when she got the call from my mother, she diverted and came straight to Bayside. Uncle Abe, Aunt Bobbie, and my cousin Shane were on their way as well. Uncle Mark (my father's brother) and Aunt Jean were coming from out of town to see my dad, too. Uncle Abe, Aunt Bobbie, and Shane said their goodbyes to my father, and after that my mom sat with my dad for a while. He had both hands tightly twisted together, and my mom had to pry his hands apart so she could hold one of them. His eyes started to water.

"Look, he's crying," my mom said, and I went over to comfort her.

Next, Aunt Jean and Uncle Mark arrived to say goodbye. My Uncle Mark was taller than my dad even though he was younger, and he went over first to say goodbye.

Aunt Jean stood behind him and waited for her turn. Aunt Jean was always very kind to us, and as she was my cousin Shannon's mother, she was like a second mother to me. She also shared the same birthday as my dad. When her turn came, Aunt Jean walked over to put her hand on my father's shoulder. The expression on her face was very sad.

Incidentally, this was the Sunday my husband had an MRI scan booked in, and it was nearing the time for him to leave. "Do you want me to cancel it and stay here with you?" he asked.

I said no. "There is nothing you can do here, might as well go ahead and get it done."

Eva wanted to stay behind with Grandma, so I left her there while Diego and I took my husband home to get his car. In the meantime, Aunt Joanne, Uncle Abe, Aunt Bobbie, Shane, Aunt Jean, and Uncle Mark went to get something for lunch, so when I got back with Diego, it was only my mom and Eva there.

My mom's sister Melissa texted me, and I told her that if they wanted to say goodbye, they should come now. So Aunt Melissa, Uncle Jon, and my cousin Quina arrived a few minutes later. Aunt Melissa walked over and put her hand on my dad's shoulder, just as Aunt Jean had. Uncle Jon and Quina said their goodbyes next.

Eva was amazed by how long Quina's hair was. After all, her light brown hair went down past her hips. Timidly, she asked me, "Can I go over and see the pretty lady with the long hair?"

"Of course you can talk to your cousin Quina," I responded, and we walked over.

"I like your hair," Eva said.

"Thank you," Quina said. "I grow it out and then cut it and donate it to Locks of Love. It's a program that uses real hair to make wigs for other children that don't have hair."

"Some kids don't have hair?" Eva asked.

"Yes, sometimes when you're sick you can lose your hair. The Locks of Love program makes wigs for kids that need them," I replied. Eva seemed curious, but I think she got what we were talking about.

Around 1 p.m., the hospice nurse came to check on my dad. She checked his vital signs and explained to us what the discoloration was on his exterior limbs. "As the body tries to conserve blood flow for the most vital organs—the heart and brain—the other limbs become discolored because they are not getting enough oxygen." She turned to my mom. "He's definitely imminent now."

My husband had just returned. I looked at him and shook my head to indicate my father's condition was not good.

I had noticed my dad was skipping some of his breaths, and his breathing had become more labored in the last few hours. My mom asked the hospice nurse, "Is there any way to know how long we have with him? Should we stay all night or go home?"

"There is no way to know how long it will be," the hospice nurse replied. "If you want to go home it's okay."

I looked over at my dad, and my heart sank. I couldn't see him breathing. "Is he breathing?" I asked the nurse.

She checked, and eventually he took a breath. "It's possible to only take a breath two times every minute and still stay alive," the nurse said. "My mother did that when she was dying, she survived for two weeks that way."

I turned back to my dad. I still didn't see him taking any more breaths.

"How are his vitals? Does he have a pulse?" I asked.

She checked. "No but I haven't been able to get a pulse on him the last few days." I saw my dad take two more breaths. The last one was very labored. The hospice nurse described the last breaths someone takes as mechanical: they're not providing oxygen to the body. Then he stopped breathing completely, and after a few minutes, the hospice nurse called the time of death around 2 p.m.

My mother lost it. "Can it be? Is he really gone?" she asked.

"Yes, Mom, he is. I'm sorry."

I tried to choke back my tears since both my kids were in the room. I had to stay strong for them, I didn't want them to see me cry. Diego was only three, so he didn't understand what was going on. From his perceptive, Grandpa had been laying in the bed for the last two weeks, so he thought it was normal for him. However, my daughter was five, and she understood exactly what was going on and that he had died. My husband held her on his lap and hugged her while I sat next to my mom and tried to comfort and calm her.

The others had not yet returned from lunch, so my mom asked me to call them and let them know my dad had died. I called Aunt Jean.

"My dad just left, he left us..." I said. "He's gone."

"I'm so sorry," she replied. "We are almost back."

I didn't call the others, which I should have, but there was a lot going on and I wasn't thinking straight. The hospice nurse came back a while later and said, "Is there anyone else coming to see him? We don't have to call the funeral home until you're ready."

"Yes," I said. "There are a few others coming, they are coming back from lunch now."

The nurse came in, hugged both my mom and me, and said, "I'm sorry. Would it be okay if I get him cleaned up?" We agreed and left the room; she was cleaning him up for when the funeral home came to get him.

Uncle Abe, Aunt Bobbie, Shane, Aunt Jean, and Uncle Mark came returned. We told them the nurse was getting my dad cleaned up for the funeral home to pick him up. Aunt Bobbie didn't realize that he had died while they were gone since I had not called her, and Aunt Jean had not told her.

While we were waiting, the hospice chaplain came by to speak to us. He was very friendly and said some comforting things. "David is in a better place now, there is no more suffering for him. Please let me know if you need anything, you can call me at any time." Once my dad was cleaned up, the relatives went in to say their final goodbyes.

While we were waiting outside Aunt Jean came up to where I was holding Eva in my arms. She saw that Eva was upset and a little confused.

"Grandpa is in heaven now," she told my daughter.

Eva responded, "In heaven?"

"Yes, he's in heaven," my mother agreed.

I let the hospice nurse know that she could call the funeral home now. After that, everyone sat in the hallway outside my father's room, and my mother and I talked about what to do for the funeral, as we had done nothing but pick out the funeral home. We didn't think my father would go downhill that fast: he was technically only in the last stage of Alzheimer's for a week. We thought we would have more time. We decided we would go to the funeral home the next day.

We left before the funeral home showed up to take my father away. I went in by myself to say goodbye one last time. I sat on the bed, trying not to break down into tears. I put my hand on his head and ran it across his hair, then hugged him.

"Goodbye, Dad."

I didn't want to leave. I wanted to stay there with him, but I knew I couldn't. I had to be strong for the kids and not break down crying. I composed myself, wiped away my tears, and headed outside.

I drove my mother home, dropped off the kids with my husband, and went back over to my mom's house until her sister Tracy arrived. My Aunt Tracy was driving from Panama City to come and stay with my mother at her house. I waited until she got there because I didn't want my mom to be alone. While we were waiting, my mom and I talked about the funeral arrangements.

"I just thought we'd have more time, I didn't expect it to happen this quick," I said.

"Yes, me either," my mom agreed. "I've already decided I want him cremated."

"I think that's a good idea, then we can take him with us in the urn, and he can be with us anytime," I said.

We had in the past few years had both our late cats cremated and put in urns. We got a black shiny cat-shaped urn for our black cat Pumma, and a glossy white cat-shaped urn for Rikku, a gray female tabby cat. I liked the idea that they were still with us at home, and if we really wanted to we could bring my father's urn around with us, like on family holidays, and he would still be near.

"Okay, I'll call the funeral home in the morning and see if I can make an appointment," I said.

"What do you think we should do for the memorial? What about having it at the church?" my mother said.

"I like that idea, and I think Dad would like it. He is the direct descendant of the church." If you remember, my great-grandfather, also named David, was the founder of the First Pentecostal Church.

A few minutes later, Aunt Tracy arrived. She was wearing a black dress with a gold necklace that had topaz-colored gemstones. She always wore the most stylish clothes and accessories, even now. Like my mother's other sisters, she looked very similar to my mom, with the same brown hair and eyes.

We said our goodbyes and I headed home.

That night, when I was putting my daughter to bed, she started crying.

"What's wrong?" I asked her, although I knew already: she was upset about her grandfather.

"I liked Grandpa, why did he have to die?" she said.

Choking back tears I responded, "Because he was old and sick."

"But I saw them give him some medicine, why didn't it help him?" she said. She was talking about the morphine: she had noticed they were coming in and giving it to him.

"There isn't any medicine to fix what Grandpa had, honey, I'm sorry," I told her.

"But they gave him medicine, I saw it!" she said.

"Yes, they did, that was to help with pain, in case he was having any. Just like when I give you Tylenol to help if you have fever or pain," I said.

She understood this but still was upset. I told her it would be okay.

"I want to hug Grandpa," she said.

"You'll be able to hug his urn after it's ready."

"What's a urn?"

"It's a container they put the ashes in once they cremate him. Remember the two cat urns we have for Rikku and Pumma our cats? It will be just like that," I said. "Okay? Go to sleep now."

Chapter Thirteen

Funeral Home

The next morning my husband and I got up and took the kids to daycare, where my daughter also attended pre-kindergarten. After that, we headed back home, and I called the funeral home, making an appointment for eleven o'clock.

I asked the funeral home if I needed to bring something for my dad to wear, and they said to go ahead and bring something even though we were doing cremation, in case we decided to do a viewing. So, my husband and I went over to my mother's house to look for something for him to wear. Most of his clothes were still at the nursing home, but he had some shirts, suits, and dress pants left at home.

I went into my father's closet with my husband to look for something. I started thinking about how it would be the last thing he was ever going to wear, and I started crying, then quickly composed myself. I picked out some black dress slacks, then looked for a shirt. He didn't have any dress shirts, but he had a lot of fishing shirts, which he loved to wear, so we decided to pick one of them.

"Let's get a long-sleeved shirt, it will hide the discoloration on his arms," I said, picking out a blue Columbia long-sleeved shirt and a white undershirt.

I looked around for shoes, but he only had one pair of tennis shoes at home. The other two pairs were at the nursing home. We had to find a shoelace for one of the shoes, then I packed the clothing in a bag. I went and looked at his collection of hats: he loved to wear ball caps. He had several extra ones from his business, so I picked a blue hat with white text that had his business name on it—Surplus and Salvage Sales, Inc.

We left for the funeral home, and Aunt Joanne met us there. It was nice to have support from Aunt Joanne, Aunt Tracy, and my husband in helping me make the hard decisions we needed to make that day.

The funeral home had a large sitting area in the front with several black and brown couches. I heard a doorbell chime when we walked in. A few seconds later an older man with graying hair came and said, "Hello, I am Dane. Are you David's family?"

"Yes," I said.

"Right this way," he said. He led us into a room with a table and six chairs. We all sat down at the table and Dane got out his clipboard with a price list.

"We want to have a cremation," I told him.

"Okay," he said, and we went over the pricing for that. It was less than I thought it would be.

"Are you going to do a memorial service?" Dane asked.

"Yes, we want to do it at the church," I said.

"And do you want David to be present at the memorial?" We wanted to have the memorial by Thursday so we decided to not have his urn there since it might not have been done in time for the funeral. It turned out to be a good choice because the urn did not come in for about a week.

"Would you like to have a viewing at the church or here?" Dane asked.

"I would like to do a viewing. How about we do it here at the funeral home?" Doing it at the funeral home was a much more cost-effective option. We didn't have to rent the casket lining they would use for the viewing, as the funeral home would put him on a gurney and cover it up with sheets. It was appropriate for a small family viewing, and that was what we wanted. We set up the viewing for Wednesday.

"Do you want to put an obituary in the paper?" Dane asked. "It's around $300 for the newspaper here, but you can write one for the funeral home website for free."

We decided we would print my dad's name and date of death in the local newspaper since that was free. We would put an actual obituary in the Panama City newspaper, and one on the funeral home website. I wrote both of the obituaries.

"Okay, we are all set on the arrangements now. Would you like to look at urns?" Dane asked.

He led us into an adjoining room. It had around five to six caskets inside, as well as a nice selection of urns. There were many in traditional shapes, in several designs or a singular color. There were several urns shaped like boxes, both marble and wood. We decided we'd like a wooden box as it reminded us all of my dad's favorite cedar box. They had several to choose from: maple, bamboo, cedar, and laminate. My father hated laminate, and my mother didn't like the bamboo, so we decided on the maple one. It was a rectangular box with a zigzag pattern around the outer edge of the lid.

"We'd like to have it engraved if this one can be," I said to Dane, as he had mentioned earlier that they could engrave most of the urns. We decided to have my father's full name, date of birth, and date of death engraved.

That afternoon we visited a florist to buy a flower arrangement for the memorial. We decided that since my dad wouldn't be present at the funeral we wanted to have a framed picture of him surrounded by flowers. They had a beautiful arrangement that would encase the framed photo. We purchased it and picked out red, white, and blue flowers.

The next day we went to the church and met with Esther, the coordinator for the memorial. Esther was very nice and extremely helpful. We discussed the schedule and what we wanted for the program, and decided on the following: the opening song would be "You Raise Me Up," which my Uncle Abe had pre-recorded. The hospice chaplain would lead the opening prayer and read the obituary I wrote for my dad. Reverend Wendell, who used to work with my dad at the store, would do the remembrances and speak about my father. My dad's longtime friend Andy would sing and play the guitar, performing "Knocking on Heaven's Door." Reverend Doug would then read the family remembrance I wrote about my dad. A pre-recorded song by my Great-aunt Shirley, "Standing In The Presence of The King," would go next, followed by my Uncle Abe singing "Amazing Grace," and then we'd end with the finishing prayer. Esther gave us some large frames that we could put additional pictures of my father in and said we could bring any remembrances of him that we wanted.

The day after that was Wednesday, the viewing at the funeral home. I decided I wouldn't let the kids come to the viewing, but I would allow them to attend the memorial since it would be just pictures of their grandpa.

We arrived ten minutes early, but they already had my dad ready, and I was happy as I was looking forward to seeing him one last time. He was lying on the gurney, draped with dark blue sheets that hung down the front, back, and sides. It looked nice; they did a good job. My father was dressed in the light blue Columbia shirt we had picked out for him, with his dark blue surplus and salvage hat. I'm fairly sure they put some makeup on him, as his skin tone was evened out and he didn't look as pale as he had been when he was dying. About fifteen people showed up for the viewing, including one of his friends from Panama City who came to say goodbye. I was happy I got there early because I got a few minutes with my dad where it was just my mother, my husband, and me. Once the viewing hour was up, everyone slowly began to leave. I felt an overwhelming urge to stay; I didn't want to leave him. I knew this was the last time I'd ever see him like this. The next time I'd see him, he'd be in the urn. After getting upset, and then composing myself, we left.

The next day was the funeral. We arrived early to set up the pictures and the few items we brought as remembrances: a few of his golf and bowling trophies, his "The Greatest Grandpa" pocket watch, and the book about his grandfather, the one who started the church we were having the funeral in, that my father loved to read. Pretty soon after that, Esther came by to check on us to see if we had everything we needed, and I told her we did.

Guests started arriving and coming to talk to us. The kids were wild, running around in circles and trying to get on the stage. I was trying to get them to calm down the best as I could. I had brought some toys because I knew they'd be bored, so they started playing toy cars with their Uncle Brian, Aunt Tracy's husband, and that calmed them down.

I let Diego watch the Nick Jr. app on my phone with the volume turned down because I knew he wouldn't sit through the memorial without something. He was really good and watched the cartoons the whole time. Eva did okay as well but kept saying, "I'm hungry," so about halfway through the memorial, I fed her some Goldfish crackers I brought with me.

After the memorial was over, the church prepared lunch for everyone that wanted to stay. They made fried chicken, mashed potatoes and gravy, green beans, corn, and rolls. They had several desserts as well, ranging from lemon cake to chocolate gateau. The food was all delicious, and they let us take a few plates home, which I thought was very nice, since it meant I didn't have to cook that night!

My husband loaded up the flowers into our van and Aunt Tracy's SUV, until both trucks were full. Once we got to my mother's house, we divided up the flowers and plants. We decided I would take the fresh-cut flowers as I am terrible with plants. I once killed a cactus by overwatering it! I do not have a green thumb as no plant so far in my care has survived. Instead, I also took the easel with my dad's picture home and put it in the living room.

While I was reheating our leftovers for dinner that night, I saw my daughter doing something out of the corner of my eye. I turned to see what it was—she was hugging the photo of Grandpa on the easel. She said, "I just wanted to hug Grandpa."

My heart went out to her. "You can go hug Grandpa as much as you want."

My son noticed, then went and hugged the photo, too. I left the picture on the easel for a while before hanging it on the wall, just so they could hug Grandpa.

Chapter Fourteen

Medicaid Application

When my dad died, his Medicaid application was still not approved, and did not come through until a month after he died. He was in the nursing home a total of four months, from November 3, 2017, to March 4, 2018. The elder law attorney, Nick, had submitted the application in November. However, we had several issues with additional documents being requested and the caseworker not being able to determine what some of the documents said—not because they were ineligible, although in one case she claimed a document was too light to read, even though Nick said he could read it perfectly fine. He had to call and explain to the caseworker what one of the bank statements said. I never met the caseworker in person, so I only know what Nick told me. Nick submitted another application right after my dad died, which was retroactive to November, and shortly after, a new caseworker was assigned to the case. One month later it was approved! Both my mother and I were so relieved that it was finally over.

A week after the memorial, the urn was ready, so my husband went to pick it up. They did a great job on the engraving; I was very pleased with its appearance.

~~~

When my dad first got diagnosed with Alzheimer's, I had a discussion with one of my friends about my father's diagnosis.

"I found out today that my dad has Alzheimer's," I said solemnly.

"I'm so sorry to hear that, my grandmother has Alzheimer's as well," he said. Their family had been dealing with the disease for some time.

"Oh, I'm sorry, I didn't know. I'm not sure what to expect. I don't know much about the disease," I said.

He told me, "Don't worry, your father won't forget you until the very end."

I felt sad upon hearing that, but since the final stage was so far off, I didn't worry about it very much at the time.
~~~

The day before my father died, when he saw Diego, he smiled, and I do believe that even though he couldn't communicate with us, he still recognized us, and he knew us until the end.

What Did You Think of **Come Home, Daddy: An Early-Onset Alzheimer's Memoir?**

First of all, thank you for purchasing this book **Come Home, Daddy: An Early-Onset Alzheimer's Memoir**. I know you could have picked any number of books to read, but you picked this book and for that I am extremely grateful.
I hope that it was enjoyable. If so, it would be really nice if you could share this book with your friends and family by posting to Facebook and Twitter. If you enjoyed this book and found some benefit in reading this, I'd like to hear from you and hope that you could take some time to post a review on Amazon.
https://www.amazon.com/gp/customer-reviews/R1QJR4P47XGNB1/ref=cm_cr_dp_d_rvw_ttl?ie=UTF8&ASIN=1720187436

Please join my mailing list at my website:

aprilenciso.com